New Trends Publishing, Inc.
401 Kings Highway
Winona Lake, IN 46590
www.NewTrendsPublishing.com
newtrends@kconline.com
US and Canadian Orders: 877.707.1776
International Orders: 574.268.2601

Available to the trade through
National Book Network: 800.462.6420

1. Menstrual cycle. 2. Natural Family Planning. 3. Fertility Awareness
4. Food and reproductive health. 5. Breastfeeding and healthy child-spacing

Printings: 5,000; 5,000; 10,000; 10,000.

The author gratefully acknowledges Avery/Penguin for permission to publish this book, which is a modified version of *The Garden of Fertility*, published by Avery/Penguin in 2004.

The author also extends hearty thanks to the people who made this book possible: some yogurt makers and several insistent farmers in Lancaster County, Pennsylvania—and a few midwives there, too; everyone who shared their story about Fertility Awareness; Betsy Amster; Barbara Moore Busko; Natalie Hill, Ilene Richman; Louise Rubin; Bianca Sopoci-Belknap; Sage Wheeler; Janna Weil; and Lena Zook.

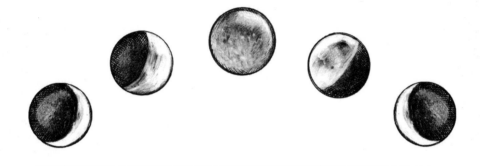

Honoring Our Cycles

A *Natural*
Family Planning Workbook

By Katie Singer

Table of Contents

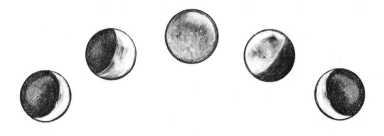

Introducing Natural Family Planning

Anyone who lives near animals knows that there are days when female animals can get pregnant and days when they can't get pregnant. All the dogs in the neighborhood know when a female dog is in heat, because she has a special smell. If you want a cow to get pregnant, you bring a bull to her when she has mucus hanging near her tail.

Gardeners know that there are good days to plant seeds—and days when it's better to wait. Usually, you want to plant after the last frost and when the moon is in a helpful phase. You want the soil moist and rich in minerals.

Everyone knows that women and men are different. Women can get pregnant. Men can't get pregnant. Also, women are *fertile* in cycles. Fertile means able to get pregnant. There are days when a woman is fertile, and there are days when she is *infertile*. Infertile means not able to get pregnant. But a man can help a woman to start a pregnancy any day. Men are fertile all the time.

In the same way that animals and the earth give signs about their fertility, a woman's body gives signs about when she can get pregnant and when she can't. Every woman can learn to read these signs, which are part of her menstrual cycle.

Farmers think about the health of a cow before they bring a bull to her, and they make sure their soil is healthy and that the weather is right before they plant a crop. We can also trust women to know when they feel strong enough for a new pregnancy and to care for a new baby.

A NATURAL SYSTEM

Natural Family Planning (NFP) is a natural system that tells women and couples when they are fertile and not fertile. It is based on charting the fertility signs that a woman's body freely gives. This system is also called *Fertility Awareness (FA)*.

A woman has four main *fertility signs*. The first sign is called *cervical mucus*. A lot of women notice this mucus on their underwear, but they don't know what it is. Mucus can keep *sperm* (the seeds from a man that are needed to start a baby) alive for up to five days.

Usually, for about ten days every cycle, a woman makes mucus that can keep sperm alive. While she has mucus, a woman is fertile and she can get pregnant. During the rest of the cycle, a woman makes no mucus. Or, she makes a kind of mucus that can't keep sperm alive.

The second sign is the woman's *vaginal sensation*. (Sensation is another word for "feeling.") If a woman charts whether the lips of her vagina feel wet or dry, then she has another way to know if she is fertile. Usually, when her vagina feels wet, she is fertile. Usually, when her vagina feels dry, she is not fertile.

The third sign is the woman's *waking temperature*. She takes her temperature before she gets out of bed every day. Before *ovulation* (when the woman has a ripe egg that can start a baby), her temperature is cooler. After ovulation, either the egg is gone or a new baby has started growing. After ovulation, a woman is infertile for the rest of that cycle.

The fourth sign is a woman's *cervix*. The cervix is the opening to the womb. It is at the top of a woman's vagina. The cervix is soft, high and open when a woman is fertile. It is firm, low and closed when she is not fertile. When a woman is breastfeeding or close to menopause, her cervix can help her know when she is fertile and not fertile.

Natural Family Planning works by charting your fertility signs every day and by knowing how to read your chart. If you want to get pregnant, you know the best days to try. If you are not ready for a new pregnancy, you know the days that you should not have intercourse.

What I have written so far is just a start. To know when you are fertile and infertile, you will need to read this book several times. You may need to talk with a Fertility Awareness teacher. You will need to chart your fertility signs for at least three menstrual cycles and pass the test at the end of this book.

MARK: Shortly after we married, my wife and I had babies born a year apart. Our family was under a lot of stress. My wife felt nervous about getting pregnant again. She knew that if she got excited, lovemaking could lead to intercourse. So, sometimes she did not want me to touch her.

Then we learned that spacing our children at least three years apart gives them a better chance of being born healthy. We read a book about Fertility Awareness. We took a class, too. After charting three cycles, we know how to tell when my wife is fertile and when she is not fertile.

It's amazing! I see that spacing our children is best for my wife's health, and it's easier financially because the children are healthier. So I can wait to have intercourse, even though we are both more interested in making love when she's fertile. But I can put my desires aside for a week or so until she is not fertile. Just because she gives me a kiss, we don't have to have intercourse. Sometimes she just wants to snuggle. I trust her if she says she is not ready for a new pregnancy yet.

She is so happy that I listen to her and respect her. Sometimes she starts our lovemaking, when before it was always me. We have also learned there are many satisfying ways to be intimate besides intercourse. Talking is at the top of the list.

---

1. The Female Reproductive System

A new *menstrual cycle* starts when a woman bleeds. The bleeding days are called the *menstrual period*. The period usually lasts three to five days. It can be longer or shorter, and many women spot a little bit of blood for some days at the end of their period.

The menstrual cycle usually lasts about a month. Some women's cycles last only 24 or 25 days. Some women's cycles last 35 or 40 days or longer. While a woman breastfeeds, she might not menstruate for several months or years.

During every menstrual cycle, a woman has infertile days and fertile days. This is like the seasons of the earth, which also have cycles. The earth is infertile during the winter, and fertile during the spring.

Every menstrual cycle starts with a hormonal message from a woman's brain to her ovaries. A *hormone* is a messenger that travels through the blood from one body part to another body part.

A woman has two *ovaries* at the top of her uterus. The ovaries hold eggs that are not full-grown. Each egg is inside a shell. Every menstrual cycle, the brain sends a hormonal message that tells about 12 eggs to grow.

While these eggs grow, they make a hormone called *estrogen*. During the first part of a menstrual cycle, estrogen tells the woman's body:

- to add a layer of fresh blood to the uterus.
- to make her cervix open, soft, and high.
- to make mucus that can keep sperm alive.
- to keep a cool temperature.

The *uterus* is a muscle. Some people call it the *womb*. The uterus is where a baby grows during pregnancy. Every menstrual cycle, estrogen tells the uterus to make a new layer of blood.

The new layer of blood inside the uterus is called the *uterine lining*. If you get pregnant, this lining will give your baby a place to start growing. If you do not get pregnant, you will bleed and let go of this lining. The bleeding is called your menstrual period.

The *cervix* is at the bottom of your uterus, and it points into your vagina. The cervix has an opening called the *os*. When you are fertile, estrogen tells your os to be soft, open, and high. Menstrual blood passes through the os. During labor, the os opens 10 centimeters (about four inches) so the baby can be born.

The cervix has little pockets; estrogen tells these pockets to make mucus. In the cervix, mucus can keep sperm alive for up to five days. Your mucus helps sperm stay alive in your cervix after you and your husband make love. Mucus also helps sperm to swim from the cervix to an egg when the egg is fully grown. Before you have a full-grown egg, your temperature is cooler.

At the top of your uterus, there are two *fallopian tubes*. Each tube has *fingers*. When one egg is fully grown (and about the size of a dot), it breaks out of its shell and out of the ovary. Right when that happens, the fingers from a tube reach for the egg and take it into the tube. The ripe egg will live in the tube for 12-24 hours. This is called *ovulation*.

If there are sperm in your cervix during ovulation, they can swim up to the fallopian tube to meet the ripe egg.

Conception happens when your husband's sperm join with the ripe egg in your fallopian tube. Conception is the start of a new baby. At this stage, the new baby is called an *embryo*. The embryo will take about a week to move down your tube and into your uterus.

Let's go back to your ovary. After ovulation (when the egg breaks out of its shell and out of your ovary), the empty shell gets a new job. Now, it makes a hormone called *progesterone*. Progesterone does many things. It:
- makes your uterine lining like a sponge.
- tells your cervix to be closed, firm, and low.
- dries your mucus and your vaginal sensation.
- warms your body temperature.

Pregnancy starts when the new baby nests in the fresh layer of blood in your uterus, about a week after conception.

If you *don't* get pregnant, then about two weeks after you ovulate, the shell will die and your temperature will drop. You will start bleeding within a day or two. A new menstrual cycle will begin.

If you *are* pregnant, the embryo will make a hormone called *HCG*. HCG tells your body to keep warm and care for the baby that you are growing. You will have 18 days of high temperatures after ovulation, and your temperature will stay warm.

Here is a drawing of the female reproductive system:

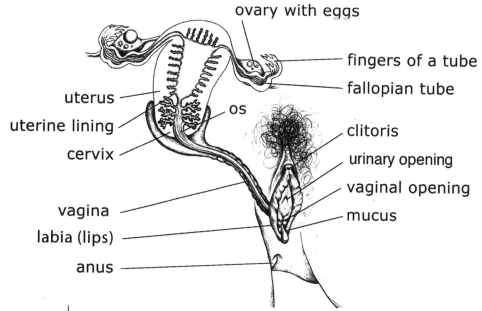

It's also important to know these parts of a woman:
The *labia* are the lips between your legs.

A woman has two small holes between her labia. The top hole is the *urinary opening*; urine comes out of this hole. The other hole goes to the *vagina*. The vagina stretches to your cervix. A man's penis enters the vagina during intercourse. A baby passes through the vagina during birth.

When a woman wants to make love, the walls of her vagina get slippery with *arousal fluid* so that intercourse will not be painful for her. Arousal fluid looks and feels like slippery mucus, but it is not the same.
Arousal fluid can not keep sperm alive.

The *clitoris* holds a woman's most sensitive nerves. The clitoris and the penis are similar in this way. The clitoris is about the size of an apple seed. It is under a small hood where the lips of the vagina come together. When a woman's clitoris is touched gently with a moist finger before intercourse, she may experience good feelings called an *orgasm*. A man experiences an orgasm when sperm come out of his penis. Some cultures believe that when a wife has an orgasm, it is also healing for her husband.

Here is a drawing of the menstrual cycle:

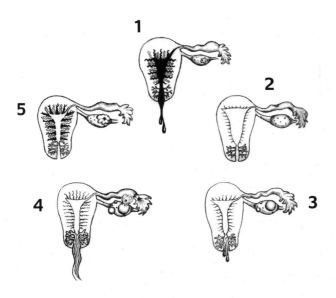

1. *The menstrual cycle starts with bleeding called a period. The period usually lasts 3-5 days.*
2. *Usually, after your period, you have no mucus, temperatures are low, and the cervix is firm and closed.*
3. *After your period (or, sometimes, during the end of your period) about 12 eggs start to grow in their shells and make estrogen. Estrogen tells your cervix to make mucus. (Mucus can keep sperm alive for up to five days). Estrogen makes your vaginal sensation wet. It cools your body temperature. It makes your cervix open, soft, and high in your vagina. Estrogen also makes a new, bloody lining in the uterus. This part of the cycle, when estrogen is strong, usually lasts about 10 days. When a woman breastfeeds, this part of the cycle can last for months or years. It can also last a long time when a woman has Poly-Cystic Ovarian Syndrome (PCOS).*
4. *When an egg is ripe, it breaks from its shell and from the ovary, and the fallopian tube's fingers take the egg into the tube. This is called ovulation. The ripe egg will live in the tube for 12-24 hours. Vaginal sensation can be very wet, and mucus can be very slippery at ovulation (like in this drawing). Sometimes mucus starts to dry up at ovulation.*
5. *After ovulation, the empty shell that held the ripe egg makes progesterone. Progesterone makes the new bloody lining in your uterus like a sponge. It dries up your mucus. It warms your body temperature. It makes your cervix firm, closed and low in the vagina. If you don't get pregnant, then the shell dies about two weeks after ovulation, and a new cycle begins. You start bleeding again. If you do get pregnant, this shell will live for three months; it will keep making progesterone to help your body care for your growing baby.*

2. How To Chart Your Fertility Signs

A woman of childbearing age has four main fertility signs: her mucus, vaginal sensation, waking temperature, and cervix changes. Every menstrual cycle, your fertility signs go through many changes. If you look at these signs every day and write them down on a chart, then you can know when you are fertile and when you are not fertile.

MUCUS

Mucus is made in the cervix. It has two main jobs:
- it feeds sperm.
- it helps sperm travel up the uterus and to the ripe egg in the fallopian tube at ovulation.

Usually, after the period, there is no mucus. You are dry. Then a bit of sticky mucus shows up for a day or two. Then you might see creamy mucus for a few days. Next, for another few days, the mucus is slippery, like eggwhite. Then the mucus dries up and stays dry until a new period starts.

You need to check your mucus three times each day. Before you check, wash your hands. Many women find it easy to check before they urinate. Take a sample of mucus by wiping the tip of your clean finger just inside your vagina. Some women prefer to take a sample of mucus with a folded square of tissue.

Feel the sample before you look at it. (If you take your sample with tissue, you still need to feel the mucus with your fingers.) Is there anything there? Sometimes, nothing's there, and you feel dry.

If you do have mucus, it might be sticky, milky, creamy, or slippery and stretchy. *Sticky* is like the paste you used in first grade. *Creamy* is like hand lotion. *Slippery* is like the *eggwhite* of an egg in your kitchen.

Your mucus might not be like these examples. Talking with a Fertility Awareness teacher can help you learn what to write on your chart.

Here is a drawing of mucus samples:

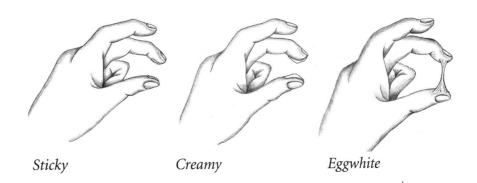

Sticky   *Creamy*   *Eggwhite*

Before you go to sleep, on your chart, write down what your mucus was like during the day. You need to write down your wettest sample. For example, if your mucus was dry in the morning, creamy at noon, and dry again in the evening, write creamy on your chart.

If you have eggwhite that stretches to two inches, write *eggwhite, 2".* Or, for shorthand, you could write *2".*

Here is an example of a mucus chart:

Cycle day	1	2	3	4	5	6	7	8	9	10	11	12	13	14	15	16	17	18	19	20	21	22	23	24	25	26	27	28	29	30	31	32	33	34	35	36	37	38	39	40	41
Mucus	medium flow	medium flow	light flow	spotting	dry	dry	dry	crumbly	sticky	creamy	creamy	eggwhite, 2"	3"	dry	dry	dry	dry	dry	dry	dry	dry	dry	dry	dry	dry	dry	new cycle														

On Day 4, this woman was spotting blood. On Days 5-7 and Days 14-26, she had no mucus, so she wrote "dry" on her chart. On Day 13, she had three inches of eggwhite. Her new cycle started on what would have been Day 27. She started a new chart on that day.

If your mucus is yellow or greenish, if it smells funny, or if it does not change from one period to the next, you might have a vaginal infection. Please see a doctor.

VAGINAL SENSATION

When you wipe yourself with tissue after urinating, you may notice that the lips of your vagina sometimes feel dry. Sometimes they feel wet. This is your vaginal sensation, your vaginal feeling. Usually, the lips to a woman's vagina feel dry after her period, wet before ovulation, and dry after ovulation.

Without touching, most of us know if the inside of our nose feels wet or dry. When you chart your vaginal sensation, you learn to know if the lips to your vagina feel wet or dry.

Please note that sometimes you can have a wet sensation and no mucus. Sometimes you can have mucus and a dry sensation.

At the end of the day, mark the wettest sensation from the day on your chart. *W* = wet or moist. *D* = dry.

Here's a chart showing mucus and vaginal sensation:

Cycle day	1	2	3	4	5	6	7	8	9	10	11	12	13	14	15	16	17	18	19	20	21	22	23	24	25	26	27	28	29	30	31	32	33	34	35	36	37	38	39	40	41
Peak Day																																									
Vaginal Sensation						D	D	W	W	W	W	W	D	D	W	W	W	W	W	D	D	D	D	D	D	D	D	D	D	D	D	D									
Mucus	heavy flow	medium flow	medium flow	medium flow	spotting	dry	dry	moist	creamy	creamy	stretchy	eggwhite. 1"	creamy	tacky	creamy	creamy	eggwhite. 1"	eggwhite. 2"	creamy, drier	tacky	dry	dry	dry	dry	dry	dry	dry	dry	dry	dry	dry	dry	new cycle								

On Day 8, this woman began feeling a wet vaginal sensation and she noticed moist mucus. On Day 13, her mucus was creamy and she had a dry vaginal sensation. On Day 19, her mucus was drier than it was on Day 18 and her vaginal sensation was still wet.

Some women's mucus does not change from day to day. It is always creamy or sticky. It is never like eggwhite. Two weeks of this kind of mucus are called a *basic infertile pattern*, or *BIP*. A BIP is common in women who do not ovulate. When a woman comes off the Pill, breastfeeds, or gets near menopause, it is common for her not to ovulate. If your mucus does not change from day to day and you have a BIP, please read pages 23-24.

THE WAKING TEMPERATURE

The waking temperature is your body's temperature before you get out of bed in the morning. Usually, a woman is cool before ovulation and warm after ovulation.

To chart your waking temperature, you need a digital thermometer with a memory. Most drug stores sell digital thermometers for about ten dollars each. (If you have an old mercury thermometer, it should measure from 96 to 100 degrees.)

- Put your thermometer on a table next to your bed.
- Take your temperature at the same time every day when you wake up. If you take it at a different time one day, mark the time on your chart.
- Take your temperature under your tongue every day.
- Take your temperature before you eat, drink, make love, urinate, have a bowel movement, or climb stairs.

The thermometer will keep a memory of the last temperature you take, so you do not need to read or chart your temperature until you go to bed.

Do your best to take your temperature at the same time every morning.

Your waking temperature can be affected by illness, restless sleep, travel, drinking alcohol the night before, sleeping with an electric blanket or on a heated waterbed, or by taking your temperature at a different time than usual. It will probably not be affected by sleeping with extra blankets or a child, or in a room that is cooler or warmer than usual. If you think your temperature was affected by one of these things—or something else—write a note to yourself on your chart.

Here is a chart of a woman's waking temperature during one menstrual cycle:

Waking Temperature	Cycle day

(Temperature chart grid showing waking temperatures plotted for cycle days 1 through 41. Temperature rows range from 96.9 up to 99.9. Circled/plotted points trace the woman's daily waking temperature across the cycle, with a thick vertical line marking the end of the cycle after day 38.)

On Day 1 (the first day of bleeding), this woman's waking temperature was 98.0. On Day 8, it was 96.9. On Days 16 and 17, it was 97.5. On Day 28, it was 98.2. She started a new cycle on what would have been Day 39. She drew a thick line to mark the end of the cycle. For her new cycle, she should get a new blank chart, and circle 97.9 for Day 1.

CERVIX CHANGES

The cervix is usually soft, open, and high in the vagina when a woman is fertile. When she is infertile, the cervix is usually firm, closed, and low.

For many women, mucus, vaginal sensation and the waking temperature give enough information to know when they are fertile and infertile. However, if you are breastfeeding, coming off the Pill or Depo-provera, or close to menopause, you may not be ovulating regularly. Charting your cervix (along with your other fertility signs) can give you helpful information.

For many women, the cervix is a mysterious part of the body. It may take a while to get used to feeling your cervix, and to get the information you need for your chart. It may help to look again at the picture on page six.

Wait until your period has ended to feel your cervix. Check once a day, at about the same time—say before or after you shower.

Wash your hands well, then squat or lift one foot on the bathtub. Put your clean middle finger (with a trimmed nail) all the way into your vagina. Your cervix might feel like the tip of your nose.

The cervix is often straight around ovulation and tipped to the right or the left on infertile days. If you squat, your cervix may be easier to feel.

You want to know your cervix's texture and location, and how open the os is.

- The texture of your cervix might feel firm, like the tip of your nose. Or, it might feel soft like your tongue.
- The cervix's location can be low, midway, or high in your vaginal canal.
- The os can be closed, partly open, or very open.

To chart your cervix's texture, use the letters *F*, *M*, and *S* to mean firm, medium, or soft. To chart your os's opening and location, mark a closed or open circle low, midway, or high on your chart.

This chart shows a woman's cervix changes during one menstrual cycle:

Cycle day	1	2	3	4	5	6	7	8	9	10	11	12	13	14	15	16	17	18	19	20	21	22	23	24	25	26	27	28	29	30	31	32	33	34	35	36	37	38	39	40	41
Cervix							•	•	•	•	o	o	o	o	O	O	•	•	•	•	•	•	•	•	•	•	•	•	•	•	•										
							F	F	F	F	M	M	M	M	S	S	F	F	F	F	F	F	F	F	F	F	F	F	F	F	F										

This woman's cervix is low, closed, and firm on Days 7-10 and Days 17-31. It is located midway in her vagina, it is a little bit open, and the texture is medium (not soft, not firm) on Days 11-14. On Days 15 and 16, her cervix is high, open and soft. Notice that she does not check her cervix on the first days of her cycle, when she is bleeding or spotting.

Becoming familiar with your cervix takes practice. If you would like to see pictures that show how the cervix changes during a cycle, go to www.GardenofFertility.com. Click on "Natural Birth Control" or "Getting Pregnant," and then click on "Cervix Pictures."

HOW TO RESEARCH YOUR OWN HEALTH

The section at the bottom of the chart (see page 16) can help you to research your own health. Some women mark their charts when they eat sugar, exercise, feel depressed, have headaches, are interested in sex, or take medication. They chart to see if any of these things might relate to their cycles.

For example, a woman who wants to see whether eating sugar affects her cycle can write "sugar" in this section and check the box every day that she eats some. Or, she could mark how much sugar she eats with a scale from one to ten. She might mark a "3" if she ate sweet pickles, a "6" if she also drank a glass of juice, and a "10" if she also ate a cookie.

TO LEARN what happens to the menstrual cycle when a woman takes birth control pills, please see page 48 .

CHARTING LINE BY LINE

Fertility Cycle #: On this line, mark the number of cycles you have charted. If this is the second cycle that you are charting, put a 2 here.

Start Date: This is the date that your menstrual period (bleeding) starts.

 # Days this cycle length: Here you mark the number of days from the start of one cycle until the last day of that cycle. For example, if you start a new period on Day 1 and the next period on what would have been Day 32, your cycle would be 31 days long.

Cycle day: Day 1 is the day your period starts. Day 2 is the second day of your cycle, and so on. When you get a new period, start counting from Day 1 again.

Date: Here you mark the date. (March 23, for example).

Intercourse: Check this box on the days you have intercourse.

Temp Count: Here, you confirm ovulation by your temperature. Pages 24-27 explain how.

Waking Temperature: In this section, mark your waking temperature.

Peak Day: This will tell you when you are fertile and infertile by your mucus and vaginal sensation. Pages 20-22 explain how.

Cervix: Marking information about your cervix takes two lines. In the top box, draw a closed or open circle to show how open your cervix is. Place this circle low, midway, or high in the box to show your cervix's location in your vagina. In the box below this circle, write an *F* if your cervix felt firm that day, *M* for medium, or *S* for soft.

Mucus: Here, after your period, write down "dry" when you see no mucus that day. When you do have mucus, write down your wettest sample from the day—sticky, creamy, or eggwhite.

Vaginal Sensation: After your period, your vaginal sensation will be dry or wet. Write down D for dry or W for wet.

BSE: BSE stands for Breast Self-Exam. Day 7 of each cycle is a good day to feel your breasts for lumps. Most lumps are not cancerous. Still, if you have a lump, get it checked by your doctor. Once you have checked your breasts, you can circle BSE on your chart.

Miscellaneous: In this section, you can research whatever you want about your health and your cycle—perhaps the days you exercise, eat sugar, feel moody, experience headaches. For example, write "yoga" on the line at the left, then check each day that you practice it.

You don't have to wait for your next period to start charting. Say your last period started ten days ago. You can check your mucus today and begin charting it today (which would be Day 10, if your period started ten days ago). Get yourself a thermometer, take your temperature on the morning of Day 11, and you're on your way.

Many women find that the hardest part of charting is getting into the habit of it. Once you're in the habit, it's easy to continue. Call a girlfriend who's also learning the method. Write down your questions about it in a diary. If you don't get answers to your questions from this book, please contact a Fertility Awareness teacher. Page 63 ("Helpful People") tells how to find a teacher.

RUTH: I never understood how my hormones change around my period and when I ovulate until I learned to chart. My girlfriends and I all have problems with our cycles. Fertility Awareness helps us ask better questions about what we can do to get healthier. We're not married, but we chart our fertility signs because we want to understand our bodies. And if we do get married, we will know how to give our families healthy child-spacing.

This chart shows all four fertility signs during one menstrual cycle:

Fertility Cycle # __9__

Start Date __March 23__   # Days this cycle __31__

Cycle day	1	2	3	4	5	6	7	8	9	10	11	12	13	14	15	16	17	18	19	20	21	22	23	24	25	26	27	28	29	30	31	32	33	34	35	36	37	38	39	40	41
Date	3/23	24	25	26	27	28	29	30	31	4/1	2	3	4	5	6	7	8	9	10	11	12	13	14	15	16	17	18	19	20	21	22										
Intercourse																																									
Time Temp Taken	6	6	6	6	6	6	6	6	6	6	6	6	6	8	6	6	6	6	6	6	6	6	6	6	9	6	6	6	6	6	6										
Temp count																																									

Waking Temperature (chart grid, 99–97)

Cycle day	1	2	3	4	5	6	7	8	9	10	11	12	13	14	15	16	17	18	19	20	21	22	23	24	25	26	27	28	29	30	31	32	33	34	35	36	37	38	39	40	41
Peak Day																																									
Vaginal Sensation							D	D	D	W	W	W	W	W	W	W	W	D	D	D	D	D	D	D																	
Cervix					•	•	•	•	•	O	O	O	O		O O		•	•	•	•	•	•	•	•																	
Cervix F/M/S					F	F	F	F	M	M	M	M	M	S	S	F	F	F	F	F	F	F																			

| Mucus | heavy flow | heavy flow | med. heavy flow | light flow | spotting | spotting | dry (BSE) | dry | slight cream | milky | milky – bouncy | milky – bouncy | creamy | creamy | slight stretch | stretchy | dry | dry | dry | dry | dry | dry | dry | dry | creamy | dry | | | | | | | | | | | | | | | | |

Cycle day	1	2	3	4	5	6	7	8	9	10	11	12	13	14	15	16	17	18	19	20	21	22	23	24	25	26	27	28	29	30	31	32	33	34	35	36	37	38	39	40	41
Miscellaneous:																																									
yoga			✓				✓				✓			✓	✓					✓				✓																	
headaches										1									8																						
sugar								5											7	4																					

This woman took her temperatures later than usual on Days 14 and 25, and she marked the times on her chart. She has not yet filled in the lines for "Temp Count" or "Peak Day." You'll learn how to fill these in on pages 20 and 24. This woman and her husband did not have intercourse during this cycle because they are learning Fertility Awareness. She marked when she did yoga, when she got headaches, and when she ate sugar. She is doing research on her menstrual cycle!

3. How To Tell When a Woman is Fertile or Infertile

A woman is fertile when she has mucus that can keep sperm alive. She is fertile in the days before she ovulates. *Ovulation* is when you have a fully grown egg in a fallopian tube. By charting your fertility signs, you can know when you are fertile and infertile each cycle. You can know whether you ovulate. In this chapter, I explain how to know the days that lovemaking can *not* lead to pregnancy. Once you know this, then learning when to make love to *get* pregnant is much easier.

DURING THE MENSTRUAL PERIOD

Most women will not get pregnant if they have intercourse during their menstrual period. However! *It is possible* to become pregnant if you have intercourse during your period. While you bleed or spot, your eggs can grow and make estrogen—and estrogen gets you to make mucus. While you bleed or spot, you can not tell if you have mucus.

Say that you have intercourse on Day 4, while you are still bleeding. It is possible that you could also start making mucus (which can keep sperm alive for up to five days) on Day 4. Menstrual blood, mucus, and sperm can all live together in your cervix. Say that you ovulate on Day 8 in this same cycle. You could have sperm ready to travel to your ripe egg—and start a pregnancy.

The only rule for knowing whether you are fertile while you bleed is based on past cycles. You need to know how long your last 12 cycles were. You also need a clear temperature shift that showed ovulation in your last cycle.

- If your last 12 cycles were all 26 days or longer, you can consider yourself infertile during your period's first five days.
- If any of your last 12 cycles were 25 days long or less, you can only consider yourself infertile during your cycle's first three days.

If you have ever had a short cycle and are not open to a pregnancy now, having intercourse during your period will be risky. Also, women who are near menopause should always consider the period possibly fertile, because hormonal changes before menopause can make you ovulate very early.

HOW VAGINAL SENSATION & MUCUS TELL YOU WHEN YOU ARE FERTILE AND INFERTILE

Usually, after her period, a woman will notice a dry vaginal sensation and no mucus for several days. Without mucus, sperm cannot live more than four hours.

Usually, after two or three dry days, you will start to notice mucus, and your vaginal sensation will get wet. Often, the mucus starts with a sticky texture, like paste. Then it turns creamy, like lotion. Then it gets slippery, like eggwhite.

Once you have any mucus *or* a wet vaginal sensation after your period, the fertile part of your cycle has started. The mucus and the wetness are signs from your body. They tell you that you can keep sperm alive and you have eggs that are getting ripe. As soon as you notice wet vaginal sensation or mucus after your period, consider yourself fertile.

Usually, mucus gets slippery like eggwhite just before ovulation, and then it dries up. Vaginal sensation will also dry up after ovulation. Usually, these will both stay dry for the rest of your cycle.

Not all cycles are like this. For example, if you have a short cycle, mucus can start to show up during the period or immediately after it.

AFTER YOUR PERIOD AND BEFORE OVULATION: THE RULES

After your period, if you have checked you mucus three times during the day (in the morning, at noon, and in the evening) and found no mucus and dry sensation each time, then you have signs from your body that you are not fertile. You do not have mucus that can keep sperm alive. After your period, if you find dry sensation and no mucus three times during the day, you are considered infertile after 6 PM of that day.

The next day, you need to check your vaginal sensation and mucus three times again. If you have no mucus and dry sensation three times during this day, you are again infertile after 6 PM.

This rule works because sperm can not live more than four hours without mucus. If you've been dry all day, and you have intercourse after 6 PM on that day, your risk of getting pregnant is less than 2%.

Here is a chart showing mucus and vaginal sensation:

Cycle day	1	2	3	4	5	6	7	8	9	10	11	12	13	14	15	16	17	18	19	20	21	22	23	24	25	26	27	28	29	30	31	32	33	34	35	36	37	38	39	40	41
Vaginal Sensation					D	D	D	D	W	W	W	W	W	W	W	D	D	D	D	D	D	D	D	D	D	D	D														
Mucus	med - heavy flow	medium flow	medium flow	light flow	dry	dry	dry	dry	dry	moist	creamy	creamy	clear. slippery 2"	tacky	dry	dry	dry	dry	dry	dry	dry	dry	dry	dry	dry	dry	new cycle														

This woman is not fertile after 6 PM on Days 5, 6, 7, and 8. The fertile part of her cycle starts on Day 9, when she notices a wet vaginal sensation. If she and her husband have intercourse while she's fertile, she could get pregnant. If they're not ready for a new pregnancy, they need to wait for intercourse until her chart says that she has ovulated. (Keep reading, and you'll learn how to do this.)

Here is another chart showing a woman's mucus and vaginal sensation:

Cycle day	1	2	3	4	5	6	7	8	9	10	11	12	13	14	15	16	17	18	19	20	21	22	23	24	25	26	27	28	29	30	31	32	33	34	35	36	37	38	39	40	41
Vaginal Sensation						D	D	D	D	W	W	W	W	W	W	W	W	D	D	D	D	D	D	D	D	D	D	D	D	D	D										
Mucus	heavy flow	heavy flow	med - heavy flow	light flow	spotting	spotting	dry	dry	slight cream	milky	milky bouncy	milky bouncy	creamy	creamy	slight stretch	stretchy	dry	dry	dry	dry	dry	dry	dry	dry	dry	dry	dry	creamy	dry	new cycle											

This woman is not fertile after 6 PM on Days 7 and 8. The fertile part of her cycle starts on Day 9, when her vaginal sensation is dry, but she notices "slight cream" mucus. If she and her husband have intercourse while she is fertile, she could get pregnant. If they are not ready for a new pregnancy, they need to wait for intercourse until her chart says that she has ovulated.

If your vaginal sensation is wet and/or if you have mucus in the days right after your period, then you do not have an infertile time before you ovulate. This can happen when a woman has short cycles.

Here is an example:

Cycle day	1	2	3	4	5	6	7	8	9	10	11	12	13	14	15	16	17	18	19	20	21	22	23	24	25	26	27	28	29	30	31	32	33	34	35	36	37	38	39	40	41
Vaginal Sensation					D	W	W	W	W	W	W	W	D	D	D	D	D	D	D	D	D	D	D	D	D																
Mucus	bleeding	bleeding	bleeding	light	spotting	spotting	creamy	creamy	creamy	slight stretch	eggwhite	eggwhite	creamy	dry	dry	dry	dry	dry	creamy	dry	dry	sticky	dry	dry	dry	new cycle															

This woman does not have any dry days after her period. She needs to consider herself fertile until she has ovulated. Note that she also has a short (25 day) cycle. For at least the next 12 cycles, she and her husband need to consider her fertile after Day 4. If they are not ready for a new pregnancy, they need to wait to have intercourse until she has been dry all day and/or until she has ovulated.

HOW TO KNOW THAT YOU HAVE OVULATED: THE PEAK DAY RULE

When your mucus gets slippery and then dries up for several days, your body has given you the sign that you have ovulated.

To notice this sign, you first have to find your *Peak Day*. The Peak Day is the *last* day of wet mucus or wet vaginal sensation. The Peak Day is not the day you have the most mucus. It is the LAST wet day before your mucus starts to dry up. You can not tell that you have had your Peak Day until the next day, when your mucus is drier than it was the day before.

Say that you have had eggwhite and wet vaginal sensation for two or three days, and then you have a day of creamy mucus with a dry sensation. The day of eggwhite would be your Peak Day, because creamy mucus is drier than eggwhite. And dry sensation is drier than wet sensation.

Do you see? When your mucus starts to dry up, you know that the day before was your Peak Day. Most women ovulate on the Peak Day.

Mark your Peak Day with a *P* on your chart. Mark the next day (when you are drier) with a #1. Mark the next day (when you are still drier) with a #2. When you have four days in a row that are drier than your Peak Day, you know that your egg for that cycle is gone. You are considered infertile after 6 PM on the fourth day.

Here is an example:

Cycle day	1	2	3	4	5	6	7	8	9	10	11	12	13	14	15	16	17	18	19	20	21	22	23	24	25	26	27	28	29	30	31	32	33	34	35	36	37	38	39	40	41
Peak Day														P	1	2	3	4																							
Vaginal Sensation						D	D	D	D	D	W	W	W	W	D	D	D	D	D	D	D	D	D	D	D	D	D	D													
Mucus	heavy flow	heavy flow	medium flow	medium flow	spotting	dry	dry	dry	tacky	tacky	lotiony	milky	eggwhite	eggwhite	creamy	tacky	dry	dry	dry	dry	dry	dry	dry	tacky	dry	dry	dry		new cycle												

This woman's Peak Day is Day 14, because it is her last day of wet mucus and wet vaginal sensation before she starts to dry up. She counts four days of mucus and vaginal sensation that are drier than her Peak Day, and then she knows that she has ovulated. In this cycle, she knows that she has ovulated by 6 PM on Day 18. She and her husband can have intercourse whenever they want during the rest of this cycle and she will not get pregnant.

Here is another example:

Cycle day	1	2	3	4	5	6	7	8	9	10	11	12	13	14	15	16	17	18	19	20	21	22	23	24	25	26	27	28	29	30	31	32	33	34	35	36	37	38	39	40	41
Peak Day															P	1	2	3	4																						
Vaginal Sensation						D	D	D	D	D	W	W	W	W	W	D	D	D	D	D	D	D	D	D	D	D	D	D													
Mucus	heavy flow	heavy flow	medium flow	medium flow	spotting	dry	dry	dry	tacky	tacky	lotiony	milky	eggwhite	eggwhite	creamy	tacky	dry	dry	dry	dry	dry	dry	dry	tacky	dry	dry	dry		new cycle												

In this cycle, the Peak Day is Day 15, because her mucus and vaginal sensation BOTH start drying up on Day 16. (On Day 15, her vaginal sensation is still wet.) After 6 PM on Day 19, this woman knows that she ovulated. She has had four days of mucus and vaginal sensation that are drier than her Peak Day. She and her husband can have intercourse as much as they like for the rest of this cycle—and she will not get pregnant because her egg for this cycle is gone.

SPLIT PEAKS

Sometimes, you may have a *"split peak."* In this case, your body gets ready to ovulate and your mucus gets wetter, but you don't ovulate. You dry up some, then start making mucus again. You know that you have not ovulated because you don't have four days that are drier than your Peak Day. Also, around your Peak Day, your temperature does not go up and stay high. (Please read the next section about how your waking temperature tells you that you have ovulated.)

With split peaks, your mucus gets wet and dries up more than once in a cycle. You might ovulate in this cycle—or you might not. Split peaks are common when women have long cycles. Women have long cycles when they breastfeed, come off the Pill, or are under stress. If you have a split peak more than once a year (and you are not breastfeeding), your charts are telling you that you may have an ovarian cyst or Poly-Cystic Ovarian Syndrome (PCOS). Please talk with your doctor and read the section about food in this book to find ways to help your cycles.

Here is an example of a chart with a split peak:

Cycle day	1	2	3	4	5	6	7	8	9	10	11	12	13	14	15	16	17	18	19	20	21	22	23	24	25	26	27	28	29	30	31	32	33	34	35	36	37	38	39	40	41
Peak Day												P	1	2				P	1	2	3	4																			
Vaginal Sensation					D	D	W	W	W	W	W	W	D	D	W	W	W	W	D	D	D	D	D	D	D	D	D	D	D	D	D										
Mucus	heavy flow	medium flow	medium flow	medium flow	spotting	dry	dry	moist	creamy	creamy	stretchy	eggwhite, 1"	creamy, dry	tacky	creamy	creamy	eggwhite, 1"	eggwhite, 1 1/2"	creamy, dry	tacky	dry	dry	dry	dry	dry	dry	dry	dry	dry	dry	dry	new cycle									

This woman's mucus and vaginal sensation are wet until Day 12, and then she starts drying up. So Day 12 is a Peak Day. But then she has wetter mucus and wet vaginal sensation starting again on Day 15. She has another Peak Day on Day 18, because her mucus and vaginal sensation start drying up on Day 19. This time, she continues to dry up. After the Peak Day on Day 18, she has four days in a row of drier mucus and drier vaginal sensation. She can consider herself infertile after 6 PM on Day 22. If her temperature also tells her that she has ovulated by Day 22, then she and her husband can have intercourse as often as they like for the rest of this cycle and she will not get pregnant.

Note that after your period and before ovulation, tacky or sticky mucus usually means that you are fertile. After ovulation, tacky or sticky mucus can mean that you are infertile—if it is drier than Peak Day mucus.

THE BASIC INFERTILE PATTERN (BIP)

If your mucus pattern does not change from dry to sticky, to creamy, to eggwhite—and then to drier mucus, you may have a hard time knowing when you are fertile and not fertile. You may not be ovulating regularly. You may feel frustrated—whether you want to get pregnant or not.

Your mucus might show what is called a *basic infertile pattern (BIP)*. With a BIP, mucus does not change from day-to-day. It is usually dry or sticky, and you do not get eggwhite. Your vaginal sensation will be dry; your temperature does not go up and stay up.

To learn your basic infertile pattern, you need to chart your mucus for two weeks. During this time, you should not have intercourse so that your husband's semen does not confuse what you see with your mucus.

Once you know your basic infertile pattern, you can apply the following two rules when you are not ready for a new pregnancy:

1. During the evening of each day that your mucus is dry or sticky (like it is in your BIP), you are not fertile.

2. If you notice a change in your BIP, find your Peak Day (the last day of wet mucus). Consider yourself fertile until the evening of the fourth day in a row of mucus that is drier than your Peak. For example, if your mucus is wet on Monday and dry on Tuesday, Monday would be your Peak Day. If you mucus stays dry Tuesday, Wednesday, Thursday, and Friday, you would be infertile Friday evening.

You can get more information by charting your cervix every day. (Please read the section about cervix changes on page 29.)

Here is an example of a BIP:

Cycle day	1	2	3	4	5	6	7	8	9	10	11	12	13	14	15	16	17	18	19	20	21	22	23	24	25	26	27	28	29	30	31	32	33	34	35	36	37	38	39	40	41
Peak Day																				P	1	2	3	4							P	1	2	3	4						
Vaginal Sensation	D	D	D	D	D	D	D	D	D	D	D	D	D	D	D	D	D	D	D	W	W	D	D	D	D	D	D	D	D	D	W	W	D	D	D	D	D	D	D	D	D
Mucus	dry	dry	dry	sticky	dry	dry	sticky	sticky	dry	sticky	dry	dry	dry	dry	sticky	dry	dry	dry	sticky	moist - creamy	sticky	dry	dry	dry	sticky	sticky	dry	dry	dry	moist	creamy - wet	sticky	sticky	dry	dry	dry	sticky	dry	sticky	dry	dry

After two weeks of dry vaginal sensation and mucus that is dry or sticky, this woman can consider herself infertile after 6 PM on Days 15-18. Her mucus and vaginal sensation get wetter than usual on Days 19 and 20. Day 20 is a Peak Day. Then she has four days in a row of mucus and vaginal sensation that are drier than her Peak Day. She is infertile again after 6 PM on Days 24-29. She has another Peak Day and again more drying up. She is infertile again after 6 PM on Days 36-41.

HOW YOUR WAKING TEMPERATURE TELLS YOU WHEN YOU ARE FERTILE AND INFERTILE

Before ovulation, your body is cooler. After ovulation, your temperature will warm up and stay warm. (Before ovulation, your eggs make estrogen, a hormone that keeps you cool and gives you wet mucus. After ovulation, the empty shell that once held your egg makes *progesterone*, a hormone that warms you up and dries your mucus.)

After ovulation, in a healthy cycle, your waking temperatures will stay warm until the shell dies and a new cycle begins. If you get pregnant, the shell will stay alive—and keep your temperature warmer—for about three months. At three months, the *placenta* takes over to make progesterone, which keeps you warm until you give birth.

Before ovulation, your temperature can not tell you if you are fertile or infertile. Before ovulation, only your mucus, vaginal sensation and cervix changes tell you when you are fertile. Still, you need to take your temperature every morning. A daily temperature chart will tell you whether you ovulate. It will also give you valuable information about your health.

CONFIRMING OVULATION BY YOUR WAKING TEMPERATURE

Day-by-day, your temperatures will go up and down a little bit. To know that you have ovulated and are no longer fertile in a cycle, you need a group of low temperatures and then a group of high ones that stay high. You need a line that separates your low temperatures (before ovulation) from your high temperatures (after ovulation). This line is called your *coverline*. To draw your coverline:

- Look for a day when your temperature jumps up.
- Put your finger on the low temperature just before your temperature jumped up.
- Starting with this low temperature before your temperature goes up, count back six temperatures.
- Find the highest of these six temperatures.
- Draw a line one tenth of a degree above the temperature that is the highest of this group of six low temperatures. This is your coverline.
- Count three temperatures in a row that are above your coverline. You are infertile after 6 PM on the evening of your third high temperature in a row above your coverline.
- Every cycle, you will need to draw a new coverline.

THE RHYTHM METHOD VS. FERTILITY AWARENESS

The Rhythm Method is based on the idea that many women start bleeding about two weeks after they ovulate.

The Rhythm Method does not work for most couples because most women's cycles are not the same every month. Illness, travel, diet, and stress can change a menstrual cycle. A woman could ovulate on Day 10 in one cycle and on Day 20 in another. While many of us expect 28-day cycles (14 days before ovulation, 14 days after ovulation), few women have such regular cycles. It is more common for a woman's cycle to change from month to month.

Because it is based on past cycles, the Rhythm Method can give you a surprise pregnancy. Or, when you want a new pregnancy, you may not know the best days to try.

With Fertility Awareness, you chart your fertility signs every day. You know how to read your chart, which tells you when you are fertile and infertile. You don't need a regular cycle to practice Fertility Awareness. You need to chart every day and to know how to read your charts.

Here is an example of a temperature chart:

Temp count														1	2	3																								
	99	99	99	99	99	99	99	99	99	99	99	99	99	99	99	99	99	99	99	99	99	99	99	99	99	99	99	99	99	99	99	99	99	99	99	99	99	99	99	99	99
	9	9	9	9	9	9	9	9	9	9	9	9	9	9	9	9	9	9	9	9	9	9	9	9	9	9	9	9	9	9	9	9	9	9	9	9	9	9	9	9	9
	8	8	8	8	8	8	8	8	8	8	8	8	8	8	8	8	8	8	8	8	8	8	8	8	8	8	8	8	8	8	8	8	8	8	8	8	8	8	8	8	8
	7	7	7	7	7	7	7	7	7	7	7	7	7	7	7	7	7	7	7	7	7	7	7	7	7	7	7	7	7	7	7	7	7	7	7	7	7	7	7	7	7
	6	6	6	6	6	6	6	6	6	6	6	6	6	6	6	6	6	6	6	6	6	6	6	6	6	6	6	6	6	6	6	6	6	6	6	6	6	6	6	6	6
	5	5	5	5	5	5	5	5	5	5	5	5	5	5	5	5	5	5	5	5	5	5	5	5	5	5	5	5	5	5	5	5	5	5	5	5	5	5	5	5	5
	4	4	4	4	4	4	4	4	4	4	4	4	4	4	4	4	4	4	4	4	4	4	4	4	4	4	4	4	4	4	4	4	4	4	4	4	4	4	4	4	4
	3	3	3	3	3	3	3	3	3	3	3	3	3	3	3	3	3	3	3	3	(3)	(3)	3	3	3	3	3	3	3	3	3	3	3	3	3	3	3	3	3	3	3
	2	2	2	2	2	2	2	(2)	2	2	2	(2)	(2)	2	2	2	(2)	2	(2)	2	2	2	(2)	2	(2)	2	(2)	2	2	2	2	2	2	2	2	2	2	2	2	2	2
	1	1	1	1	1	1	1	1	1	1	1	(1)	(1)	1	1	(1)	1	1	1	1	(1)	1	1	(1)	1	(1)	1	1	1	1	1	1	1	1	1	1	1	1	1	1	1
Waking Temperature	98	98	98	98	98	98	98	98	98	98	98	98	98	98	98	(98)	98	98	98	98	98	98	98	98	98	98	98	98	98	98	98	98	98	98	98	98	98	98	98	98	98
	9	9	9	9	9	9	9	9	9	9	9	9	9	9	9	9	9	9	9	9	9	9	9	9	9	9	9	9	9	9	9	9	9	9	9	9	9	9	9	9	9
	8	8	8	8	8	8	8	(8)	8	8	8	7	8	8	8	8	8	8	8	8	8	8	8	8	8	8	8	(8)	8	8	8	8	8	8	8	8	8	8	8	8	8
	7	7	(7)	(7)	7	7	7	7	7	(7)	7	7	7	7	7	7	7	7	7	7	7	7	7	7	7	7	7	7	7	7	7	7	7	7	7	7	7	7	7	7	7
	(6)	6	6	6	6	(6)	6	6	6	6	(6)	(6)	6	6	6	6	6	6	6	6	6	6	6	6	6	6	6	6	6	6	6	6	6	6	6	6	6	6	6	6	6
	5	(5)	5	5	5	5	(5)	5	5	5	5	5	5	5	5	5	5	5	5	5	5	5	5	5	5	5	5	5	5	5	5	5	5	5	5	5	5	5	5	5	5
	4	4	4	4	(4)	4	4	4	4	4	4	4	(4)	4	4	4	4	4	4	4	4	4	4	4	4	4	4	4	4	4	4	4	4	4	4	4	4	4	4	4	4
	3	3	3	3	3	3	3	3	3	3	3	3	3	3	3	3	3	3	3	3	3	3	3	3	3	3	3	3	3	3	3	3	3	3	3	3	3	3	3	3	3
	2	2	2	2	2	2	2	**6**	**5**	**4**	**3**	**2**	**1**	2	2	2	2	2	2	2	2	2	2	2	2	2	2	2	2	2	2	2	2	2	2	2	2	2	2	2	2
	1	1	1	1	1	1	1	1	1	1	1	1	1	1	1	1	1	1	1	1	1	1	1	1	1	1	1	1	1	1	1	1	1	1	1	1	1	1	1	1	1
	97	97	97	97	97	97	97	97	97	97	97	97	97	97	97	97	97	97	97	97	97	97	97	97	97	97	97	97	97	97	97	97	97	97	97	97	97	97	97	97	97
	9	9	9	9	9	9	9	9	9	9	9	9	9	9	9	9	9	9	9	9	9	9	9	9	9	9	9	9	9	9	9	9	9	9	9	9	9	9	9	9	9
Cycle day	1	2	3	4	5	6	7	8	9	10	11	12	13	14	15	16	17	18	19	20	21	22	23	24	25	26	27	28	29	30	31	32	33	34	35	36	37	38	39	40	41

This woman's temperature goes up on Day 14. To draw her coverline,
- *Put your finger on her temperature on Day 13 (the day before her temperature goes up).*
- *Starting with Day 13 (her last low temperature), count back six (to Day 8).*
- *The highest of these six low temperatures is 97.8 degrees.*
- *She draws her coverline at 97.9 degrees, because it is one tenth of a degree higher than 97.8*

To know when the infertile part of your cycle starts, you need to count three temperatures in a row above the coverline. Here, Days 14, 15 and 16 are above the line. This woman's after-ovulation infertile time starts on Day 16, after 6 PM. She and her husband can have intercourse as often as they want for the rest of this cycle and she will not get pregnant.

WAKING LATE, WAKING EARLY
If you take your temperature at a different time than usual (say you sleep late, or wake early), mark the unusual time on your chart. Marking the time on your chart could help explain a temperature that's different from the rest. However, if you have any doubt, consider yourself fertile.

Here is another example:

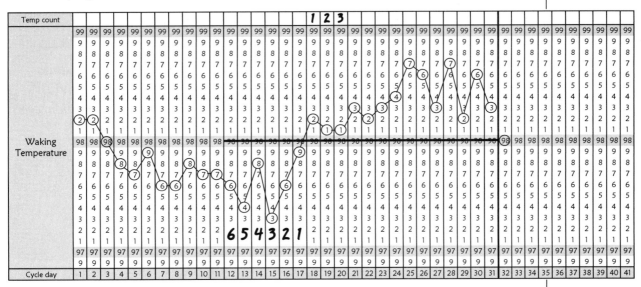

This is a tricky chart. Her temperature jumps up on Day 14. If you start counting back six temperatures on Day 13 and draw a coverline at 97.9 degrees (one tenth of a degree above the highest of the six low temperatures), then Days 15 and 16 fall below the line, and Day 17 falls right on it.

Let's try again with the same chart:

Her temperature goes up on Day 18. Put your finger on Day 17, and start counting back six temperatures. Find the highest of these temperatures (97.9). Draw a line at 98.0 degrees (one tenth of a degree higher than 97.9). Days 18, 19, and 20 are above the line! On Day 20, after 6 PM, she knows that she has ovulated. She and her husband can have intercourse as often as they like for the rest of this cycle and she will not get pregnant.

Mucus and temperature patterns don't always line up exactly. If yours do not match and you are not ready for a new pregnancy, wait to have intercourse until all off your fertility signs tell you that you are not fertile.

HOW YOUR CHART TELLS YOU THAT YOU ARE PREGNANT

Usually, there are about two weeks after ovulation, and then a new menstrual cycle begins. If you have 18 days of high temperatures after ovulating (18 temperatures above your coverline) and no period, you are probably pregnant.

Here is a pregnant woman's chart:

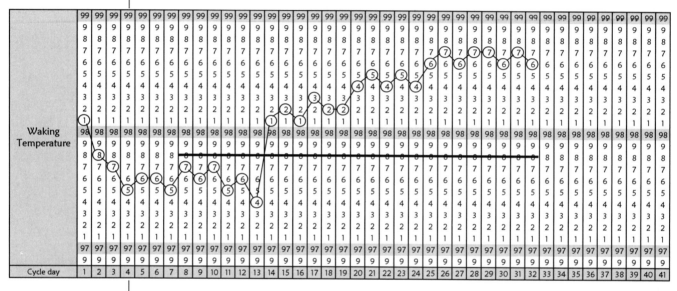

This woman knows that she is pregnant on Day 31, because she has 18 temperatures above her coverline. If her temperature dropped and she started bleeding on (say) Day 33, she would know that she probably had a miscarriage. Note that after ovulation, every five to six days, her temperature goes up a bit. This is common with pregnancy.

HOW YOUR CERVIX TELLS YOU WHEN YOU ARE FERTILE AND INFERTILE

Most of the time, charting your cervix is not necessary. But when you are breastfeeding, having problems getting pregnant, near menopause, or coming off the Pill, this sign can be very helpful.

When you are fertile, your cervix is soft and high in your vagina, and the os is open. When you are not fertile, your cervix is firm and lower in your vagina; and the os is closed.

Scientists have not studied the cervix enough to make rules about it for preventing pregnancy. But some women think that the last day that the cervix is soft, high, and open is like a Peak Day. They wait for their cervix to be firm, low, and closed for four days before they consider themselves infertile.

Here is an example:

Cycle day	1	2	3	4	5	6	7	8	9	10	11	12	13	14	15	16	17	18	19	20	21	22	23	24	25	26	27	28	29	30	31	32	33	34	35	36	37	38	39	40	41
Peak Day																P	1	2	3	4																					
Cervix (• o O / F M S)							•	•	•	•	o	o	o	o	O	O	•	•	•	•	•	•	•	•	•	•	•	•	•	•	•										
							F	F	F	F	M	M	M	M	S	S	F	F	F	F	F	F	F	F	F	F	F	F	F	F	F										

The last day that this woman's cervix is soft, high, and open is Day 16, so she marks a P on her chart. Her cervix is firmer, lower, and more closed than it was on her Peak Day for four days in a row; on Day 20, she considers herself infertile after 6 PM.

POINTS TO REMEMBER

- A woman who has mucus and/or wet vaginal sensation is fertile because her mucus can keep her husband's sperm alive until she ovulates.
- If a couple has intercourse on a Monday when the woman has mucus, and the woman ovulates five days later on Friday, her mucus can help sperm travel to her ripe egg on that Friday—and start a new pregnancy.
- If you decide when to make love based on when you ovulated in your last few cycles, you might get a surprise. Remember, every cycle is new.
- When in doubt, consider yourself fertile.

Here is chart that includes all four fertility signs:

Cycle day	1	2	3	4	5	6	7	8	9	10	11	12	13	14	15	16	17	18	19	20	21	22	23	24	25	26	27	28	29	30	31	32	33	34	35	36	37	38	39	40	41
Intercourse																																									
Temp count													1	2	3																										

(The "Waking Temperature" section is a plotted temperature graph ranging from 97.9 to 99.9, with the coverline at 98.1.)

Cycle day	1	2	3	4	5	6	7	8	9	10	11	12	13	14	15	16	17	18	19	20	21	22	23	24	25	26	27	28	29	30	31	32	33	34	35	36	37	38	39	40	41
Peak Day												P	1	2	3	4																									
Vaginal Sensation					D	D	D	W	W	W	W	W	D	D	D	D	D	D	D	D	D	D	D	D	D	D															
Cervix (F M S)					F	F	F	F	M	M	S	S	F	F	F	F	F	F	F	F	F	F	F	F	F	F															

Mucus:
- Day 1: med – heavy flow
- Day 2: med – heavy flow
- Day 3: medium flow
- Day 4: light flow
- Day 5: dry
- Day 6: dry
- Day 7: moist
- Day 8: moist
- Day 9: moist. creamy
- Day 10: creamy
- Day 11: clear. stretchy
- Day 12: 1" eggwhite
- Day 13: creamy, drier
- Day 14: tacky, dry
- Day 15: dry
- Day 16: dry
- Day 17: dry
- Day 18: dry
- Day 19: dry
- Day 20: went to sleep mad!
- Day 21: dry
- Day 22: dry
- Day 23: dry
- Day 24: dry
- Day 25: dry
- Day 26: dry
- Day 27: new cycle

This woman is infertile after 6 PM on Days 5 and 6. The fertile part of her cycle starts on Day 7, because she has moist mucus. Her Peak Day is Day 12 because it is her last day of wetness before her mucus and vaginal sensation start to dry up. Her mucus gives the sign that she has ovulated and that she is infertile for the rest of this cycle on Day 16, after 6 PM. Her coverline is at 98.1. By her temperature, she is infertile starting on Day 15 after 6 PM, because she has three temperatures in a row above her coverline on Day 15.

If she and her husband are not ready for a new pregnancy, they should wait to have intercourse until Day 16 after 6 PM, when this woman's mucus and temperature signs say that she is not fertile.

A SUMMARY OF RULES FOR NOT GETTING PREGNANT
During the Menstrual Period
Because you can have mucus while you bleed or spot (and not be able to see or feel it), consider your period a fertile time during your first 12 charted cycles. Once you have had 12 ovulatory cycles in a row that are each 26 days or longer, you can consider yourself infertile Days 1 through 5. If you have had a cycle that is 25 days or shorter, you can consider yourself infertile Days 1 through 3.

Dry Day Rule
In a dry vagina, sperm can not live more than four hours. Once you notice mucus or wet vaginal sensation, you are fertile. Intercourse can lead to pregnancy. After the period (and before ovulation), you are infertile after 6 PM if you have been dry all day. The next day, you need to be dry all day again to call yourself infertile after 6 PM.

Peak Day Rule
The last day of wet mucus or wet vaginal sensation is called the Peak Day. Women usually ovulate on the Peak Day. When your mucus has dried up for several days, you have a sign from your body that your egg is gone for this cycle. You are infertile after 6 PM when you have four days in a row of mucus and vaginal sensation that are drier than your Peak Day.

Temperature Shift Rule
When your temperature goes up, count back six low temperatures; draw a coverline one tenth of a degree above the highest of these low temperatures. When your temperature is above your coverline for three days in a row, you are infertile after 6 PM on that third day.

If You Are Not Sure Whether You Are Fertile or Infertile
If you do not want a new pregnancy and you are not sure whether you are fertile or infertile, don't have intercourse. Consider yourself fertile until all of your signs tell you that you are infertile. If your mucus and temperature do not match, listen to the one that tells you that you are still fertile.

If you are not clear about these rules, read this book again. Call a Fertility Awareness teacher. If you are not sure about when you are fertile and you are not ready for a new pregnancy, don't take the risk.

JANE, MIDWIFE: My husband and I used Natural Family Planning to space our children, and it worked beautifully for us. But as a midwife, I've seen that this method does not work for every couple. Some folks don't chart every day, and this method will not work if you do it only part of the way. A lot of mothers use pacifiers and wean their babies early, which can make pregnancies come close together. Some couples don't learn Fertility Awareness until the woman is in her late 30s or early 40s. By that age, a woman can still be fertile, but her mucus and temperature can be harder to read. At any age, if the couple does not have clear communication, the method is not reliable.

People who want healthy child-spacing need to make a commitment to charting. They need to meet with a Fertility Awareness teacher two or three times.

If Fertility Awareness is not right for a couple, then I recommend using condoms. I know that many people don't like them. But they give you a way to space your children without using drugs, and that helps your whole family to be healthier. It may take time to get used to condoms, but I think they are a good choice. When condoms are used, the woman's vagina needs to be slippery so that intercourse is not painful for her and the condom does not break. You can buy lubricant at a drug store to make the woman's vagina slippery. Do not use vegetable oil as a lubricant, because it will break the condom.

LAURA: A while ago I told my husband, "I can't have another baby." He did not understand. He said, "But the Lord only gives us what we can provide for." It was a very frustrating time in our marriage. Whenever my husband wanted to make love, I just couldn't. I felt too afraid of getting pregnant again.

We asked our midwife for help. She noticed that God has given me feelings of wanting children many times. Now, He gives me feelings that tell me I'm not ready for a new baby. She also explained that the Lord gives my body signs that tell me when I'm fertile and when I'm infertile. She showed us a book about Fertility Awareness.

My husband and I both read this book. We decided to chart my cycles, and we met twice with a Fertility Awareness teacher to make sure we understand my charts.

We have been married 20 years. Some days, while we learn about my cycles and get to know each other in new ways, I feel like we are courting again. I'm over 40, and my cycles are not regular. There have been several months that we can't tell when I'm fertile. But our communication is strong. We have also found new ways to make love without intercourse, like massaging each other. (Our midwife suggested keeping coconut oil next to the bed.)

My husband and I feel that Fertility Awareness is a blessing from God. We would like our daughters—and our sons—to learn it before they marry.

4. How Natural Family Planning Can Help You Get Pregnant

To get pregnant, you need the same information as you do when you do not want to get pregnant. You need to know when you are fertile and when you are not fertile. But now you enjoy intercourse when you are fertile.

FERTILE SIGNS: MUCUS AND VAGINAL SENSATION

Mucus and vaginal sensation give the best signs about when you are fertile and when you are about to ovulate. Remember that *being fertile* means you have mucus that can keep sperm alive. *Ovulation* is when you have a ripe egg in your fallopian tube; the ripe egg will live for 12-24 hours.

Let me also remind you about the *Peak Day*. The Peak Day is the *last* day of wet mucus or wet vaginal sensation before you start to dry up, and it tells you that you are about to ovulate. Often, a woman has eggwhite on her Peak Day.

Some women do not make mucus that is like eggwhite. Still, the last day of wet mucus or wet vaginal sensation is the Peak Day.

THE WOMAN'S FERTILITY, THE MAN'S SPERM COUNT, AND TIMING

Each menstrual cycle, a woman usually has slippery mucus for two to four days, and she has one ripe egg at ovulation. (About 10% of the time, a woman has two eggs at ovulation.)

After a man *ejaculates* (releases seminal fluid), he needs 36 hours to prepare a good amount of new sperm. A man actually needs millions of sperm to help his wife's one egg start a pregnancy.

Once you know when you are fertile and about to ovulate, you can time intercourse to help you get pregnant. If your husband has a normal sperm count, have intercourse *once each day* that you have wet mucus and wet vaginal sensation until you ovulate. If your husband's sperm count is low, have intercourse *every other day* that you have wet mucus and wet vaginal sensation.

Whether your husband's sperm count is normal or low, try to have intercourse on your Peak Day, since the Peak Day usually occurs on the day that you ovulate. This is tricky of course, because you don't know which day is your Peak Day until it has passed and your mucus has started to dry up.

If you have healthy charts but you have not gotten pregnant after a year or two of trying, you and your husband might talk to a doctor about having his sperm count tested. If your husband's sperm count is low, he should have it tested again in a few weeks, because it is common for sperm counts to be low sometimes—and then get normal again.

What can make sperm counts low? Bathing in very hot water, bicycling, tight pants, working all day near a hot oven, smoking marijuana, environmental toxins (such as pesticides), bad nutrition, soy foods, and getting older.

This chart of mucus and vaginal sensation shows a couple that is trying to get pregnant:

Cycle day	1	2	3	4	5	6	7	8	9	10	11	12	13	14	15	16	17	18	19	20	21	22	23	24	25	26	27	28	29	30	31	32	33	34	35	36	37	38	39	40	41
Peak Day																P	1	2	3	4																					
Intercourse										✓			✓	✓	✓	✓																									
Vaginal Sensation						D	D	D	D	W	W	W	W	W	W	W	D	D	D	D	D	D	D	D	D	D	D	D	D	D	D	D									
Mucus	heavy flow	heavy flow	med – heavy flow	light flow	spotting	spotting	dry	dry	slight cream	milky	milky bouncy	milky bouncy	creamy	creamy	slight stretch	stretchy	dry	dry	dry	dry	dry	dry	dry	dry	dry	dry	dry	creamy	dry	dry	dry										

This woman's Peak is Day 16. Her husband's sperm count is normal. Their best days to try getting pregnant start on Day 10, when she first notices mucus and wet vaginal sensation. Their very best days to try are Days 15 and 16, when she has eggwhite.

Here is another example. This woman's husband has a low sperm count:

Cycle day	1	2	3	4	5	6	7	8	9	10	11	12	13	14	15	16	17	18	19	20	21	22	23	24	25	26	27	28	29	30	31	32	33	34	35	36	37	38	39	40	41
Peak Day														P	1	2	3	4																							
Intercourse										✓		✓		✓																											
Vaginal Sensation					D	D	D	D	D	W	W	W	W	W	W	D	D	D	D	D	D	D	D	D	D	D	D	D	D												
Mucus	med - heavy flow	medium flow	medium flow	light	dry	dry	dry	dry	dry	moist	creamy	creamy	clear. slippery	2"	tacky	dry	dry	dry	dry	dry	dry	dry	dry	dry	dry	dry	dry	dry	dry												

This woman's Peak Day is on Day 14. Her husband's sperm count is low. Their best days to try start on Day 10, when she has wet mucus and wet vaginal sensation; their very best days to try are Days 10, 12 and 14.

I know a couple who had trouble getting pregnant. They decided to make love every other day while the woman was fertile—and she got pregnant!

SPLIT PEAKS

Sometimes, a woman will get *split peaks*. Her mucus gets wet, then dries up—but she does not ovulate. Her temperature does not jump up with the wetness on her "false" Peak Day. Then her mucus and vaginal sensation get slippery again. It might take several more false Peaks before she ovulates, or she might not ovulate for a long time.

If you have a split peak, read the food chapter. Read about night lighting on pages 50-51. Take steps to make your cycles healthier. You can also keep making love every day or every other day (depending on your husband's sperm count) when your mucus is wet. The best days to try are when you have eggwhite.

Here is an example:

Cycle day	1	2	3	4	5	6	7	8	9	10	11	12	13	14	15	16	17	18	19	20	21	22	23	24	25	26	27	28	29	30	31	32	33	34	35	36	37	38	39	40	41
Intercourse										✓		✓				✓		✓																							
Peak Day												P	1	2				P	1	2	3	4																			
Vaginal Sensation						D	D	D	W	W	W	W	D	D	W	W	W	W	D	D	D	D	D	D	D	D	D	D	D	D	D	D	D								
Mucus	heavy flow	medium flow	medium flow	medium flow	spotting	dry	dry	moist	creamy	creamy	stretchy	eggwhite 1"	creamy, dry	tacky	creamy	creamy	eggwhite 1"	eggwhite 1 1/2"	creamy, dry	tacky	dry	dry	dry	dry	dry	dry	dry	dry	dry	dry	dry	dry	dry								

This woman has a false Peak Day on Day 12; her true Peak Day is on Day 18. Her husband's sperm count is normal. Their best days to try start on Day 9 when she first notices wet mucus and wet vaginal sensation. Their very best days to try are Days 11, 12, 17 and 18.

If your mucus never gets slippery, try some experiments: stop eating sugar and white flour. Take a spoonful of cod liver every day and eat organic butter. Eat more fresh vegetables. Try sleeping in complete darkness (except for two or three days around ovulation).

THE WAKING TEMPERATURE

On the day of ovulation, a woman's temperature often dips lower. If you see this pattern in your chart, have intercourse on that day.

If you get pregnant, you will have 18 days of high temperatures above your coverline.

If you do not get pregnant, a new menstrual cycle will start about two weeks after ovulation. Your temperature will drop, and your period will begin.

BRENDA: In the first cycle we started trying to get pregnant, I got a bladder infection just before I ovulated. I told my husband, "I don't care if making love hurts—I want a baby!" As soon as I heard myself say this, I thought, "Is this how I want to invite a child into our lives?"

In fact, it is not. I have started to think that this bladder infection is my body's way of helping me slow down, be gentle with myself, and let go of the idea that I can control my body or when I get pregnant.

Here is a temperature chart from a woman who is trying to get pregnant:

Intercourse				✓				✓		✓					✓																										

Waking Temperature chart, Cycle day 1–41. Temperatures dip at Day 13 and rise above the coverline afterward.

This woman's temperature dipped lower on Day 13, when she probably ovulated. She and her husband had intercourse on Day 13. On Day 31, she knew she was pregnant because she had 18 temperatures above her coverline.

You can also have intercourse in the morning that your temperature jumps up, even though you have probably already ovulated, because there is a chance that your egg is still alive.

CERVIX CHANGES

Charting your cervix's changes gives you more information about when you are fertile and near ovulation. Usually, the cervix is soft and high and your os is open when you are fertile. It often turns firm, low in the vaginal canal, and closed just before ovulation.

To get pregnant, enjoy intercourse when your cervix gives you the signs that you are fertile.

Here is an example:

Cycle day	1	2	3	4	5	6	7	8	9	10	11	12	13	14	15	16	17	18	19	20	21	22	23	24	25	26	27	28	29	30	31	32	33	34	35	36	37	38	39	40	41
Cervix	●o O						o	o	o	O		●	o		●		o	● ●	O	● ● ●					O O		o	●	●	●	●	●	●	●							
	F M S									S		F	M				S		M			F		S	S F	F	F	F	F	F	F								

This woman's cervix is soft, high and open on Days 25 and 26. To get pregnant, she and her husband should try on those days.

I know couples who did not get pregnant for several cycles because they only had intercourse on days that the woman was not fertile. To get pregnant, you need to have intercourse when the woman has wet mucus and wet vaginal sensation!

Here is an example:

Cycle day	1	2	3	4	5	6	7	8	9	10	11	12	13	14	15	16	17	18	19	20	21	22	23	24	25	26	27	28	29	30	31	32	33	34	35	36	37	38	39	40	41
Temp Count																																									
Intercourse													✓		✓	✓																									
Peak Day																P	1	2	3	4																					
Vaginal Sensation							D	D	W	W	W	W	W	W	W	W	D	D	D	D	D	D	D	D	D	D	D	D	D	D											

Waking Temperature grid (°F), with the coverline drawn across 98 from day 12 onward; charted points rise from the mid-6s/7s in the low-98 range early in the cycle up into the 98.4–98.7 range after the rise.

Mucus row:

Day	Description
1	heavy flow
2	heavy flow
3	med – heavy flow
4	light flow
5	spotting
6	spotting
7	dry
8	dry
9	slight cream
10	milky
11	milky bouncy
12	milky bouncy
13	creamy
14	creamy
15	slight stretch
16	stretchy
17	dry
18	dry
19	dry
20	dry
21	dry
22	dry
23	dry
24	dry
25	dry
26	dry
27	dry
28	slightly creamy
29	dry
30	dry
37	pregnant!

This couple started trying on Day 13, after the woman had wetness for several days. The man's sperm count is low. They knew she was pregnant on Day 35, when she had 18 temperatures above her coverline.

YOUR DUE DATE

Doctors usually predict your due date by subtracting three months from the first day of your last menstrual period, and adding seven days. With this system, the doctor assumes that you ovulated on Day 14 of your cycle. With this system, if your last period started on January 1, your due date would be October 8.

To predict your due date by when you ovulated, subtract seven days from the first day that your temperature jumped above your coverline, then add nine months. For example, if your last period started on January 1, but you did not ovulate (and show a high temperature) until January 25, your due date would be October 18.

INFERTILITY

When a woman does not get pregnant even though her charts look healthy and she and her husband enjoy intercourse on fertile days, remember that we can not control our fertility. We can not control nature. Even when we know a lot about our bodies, getting pregnant is really a great mystery.

Not getting pregnant easily can be very painful for the husband and the wife. It raises questions about the meaning of life.

When a couple has problems getting pregnant, 40% of the time it's because of a health problem with the woman; 40% of the time it's because of a health problem with the man; and 20% of the time it's because of the couple's combined fertility.

Some people think of infertility as an opportunity to give thanks for what is good in their lives. They eat as well as they can and they exercise.

Some men and women like to talk about their experience. Some find that writing in a diary gives them comfort.

Here are some more ideas that have helped other people:

- Start a group for people in your community who have had a hard time getting pregnant. You can share your experience and ideas.
- Ask your grandparents if anyone in your family had a miscarriage, a stillbirth, an abortion, an adopted baby or infertility. These stories might help you understand your family and your place in it more fully.
- Imagine a couple you know that wants a baby. They have not gotten pregnant in two years. Or maybe the woman has had several miscarriages. They are heartbroken, and they do not know where to turn for comfort. What advice would you give this couple? Write down your advice—and consider it your best medicine.

DR. LEAH MORTON:
Some couples expect to get pregnant right away once they start trying. I think this comes from our culture's idea that we can and should control our lives. But really, we can't control our fertility. We CAN be aware of it.

If a couple has difficulty getting pregnant or keeping a pregnancy, my first concern is with their diet. Eating healthy food is one of the hardest things to do in our culture. It also makes for healthier parenting!

FERTILITY DRUGS AND TREATMENTS

Fertility drugs like Clomid work by tricking the body into making more and more hormones that cause more unripe eggs to grow than normal. These unripe eggs get a woman's body to make more estrogen than she does without Clomid. This could be a problem, because some scientists have found that the more a woman is exposed to estrogen, the more she is at risk of getting cancer.

In vitro fertilization (IVF) is a medical treatment that starts the baby outside of a woman's body.

Fertility drugs and in vitro fertilization can increase a woman's risk of ovarian cancer and her children's risk of birth defects. Also, Clomid can dry up mucus, which makes it difficult for sperm to reach mature eggs.

Fertility drugs and treatments have helped some couples to get pregnant, but they are not right for everyone. There are alternatives. Learning Fertility Awareness is a great start. Eating well is another.

ANNIE: I rarely had periods when I was a teenager. When I was 17, one of my ovaries was removed, but that did not help anything. My cycles usually last three or four months now, and I still get strong cramps for four or five days before my period starts and for the first few days that I bleed. I have been married two years, and I have not been able to get pregnant.

Two of my friends just had miscarriages—one for the second time. I know three couples who can't have children because the husband's sperm count is so low. My friends are all in their twenties, like me.

I really wonder what causes these problems, and what could make us healthy. When my mother was our age, she only knew one couple who could not have children. My friends and I feel so uninformed. Many of us grew up on farms that were regularly sprayed with pesticides and chemical fertilizers. We drank milk and ate meat from cows that were given antibiotics and bovine growth hormones. Did this affect our fertility?

I know an organic farmer who goes to my church. If I start buying our food from him, will my health get better? How long will it take to notice a difference?

I have so many questions. I read books about nutrition, organic gardening, and Fertility Awareness. I go to a fertility doctor, but he has only offered me expensive drugs. I am going to read about these drugs at the library before I decide to take them or not.

I talk with my friends and family about my concerns. Slowly—very slowly—I am changing what my husband and I eat.

I face the possibility that I might not be able to have children of my own. My husband knew about my problems before we married, but this is still so hard. He loves children, and I ache that I have not been able to give him any.

I also find myself thankful for my parents, my husband, and even my curiosity. I have never been interested in cooking, but I want to become healthy so much that I have started to read cookbooks and try new recipes.

BERNICE: I married late in life. I thought I could not get pregnant because of my age. But I did get pregnant when I was 42. I miscarried at six weeks. After the miscarriage, I brought my charts to my doctor. He could tell from my charts that I was fine. Then he asked if I wanted fertility tests.

I asked him if it is harder to get pregnant or keep pregnant. He said that at my age, getting pregnant is harder. Well, I had just done that. So I decided not to take the tests. I decided I did not want Clomid, either, after I read that this drug can increase a woman's risk of ovarian cancer. My mother died of ovarian cancer.

I got pregnant with our daughter a few months after the miscarriage. She is nine years old now—and wonderful!

A SUMMARY OF WAYS TO HELP YOU GET PREGNANT

1. If your husband's sperm count is normal, have intercourse each day you have wet mucus or wet vaginal sensation. If his sperm count is low, have intercourse every other day that you have wetness. Either way, try to have intercourse on your Peak Day.

2. Have intercourse on the first morning that your temperature jumps up.

3. Eat a healthy diet. (Read Chapter 7, which starts on page 52.) Exercise regularly. Sleep in total darkness except around the days you have slippery mucus. (Read more about night lighting on pages 50-51.)

5. Fertility Awareness While Breastfeeding

For the health of a mother, her children, and a whole family, spacing children at least three years apart is best. The mother can stay healthy and keep good energy. She has time to build up her nutrition before she starts a new pregnancy, so every child has a good chance of being born healthy. Also, every child can get good attention from Mom and Dad when they need it.

How does a couple space their children? They know when the wife is fertile, and they do not have intercourse on those days. Also, the mother breastfeeds!

In the first month after birth, the mother gives her attention to creating a healthy breastfeeding relationship with her new baby. She nurses once or twice every hour during the day and two or three times each night. She carries her baby in a sling for easy nursing. She never gives her baby pacifiers.

When a woman breastfeeds in this way, her mucus usually gets dry and stays dry. She knows that she is not fertile because she does not have wet mucus and she is not ovulating. When she sees wet mucus again, her body has given the sign that her fertile cycles are coming back—and she needs to start charting again.

HERE ARE THINGS YOU CAN DO TO SPACE YOUR CHILDREN:
- *In your baby's first few months, let him nurse once or twice every hour.* A feeding might last for 20 minutes or longer. Or, it might last 30

seconds. Your baby might want to nurse right after the last feeding. Or, he might wait to nurse again for an hour. Babies do not feel hungry on a schedule. They need to nurse when they are hungry or hurting. Nursing your baby when he cries a little bit (or lets you know in some other way that he needs to nurse) is called *nursing on cue*.

- *Nurse two or three times at night.* When your baby sleeps with you or her crib is right next to your bed, you don't need to get out of bed to nurse. Families who sleep like this can get good rest. When a baby sleeps through the night, the mother's milk might dry up. Also, the mother can become fertile again more quickly.
- *Sleep in complete darkness.*
- *Wear your baby in a sling.* He can nurse as often as he wants, and you can keep doing your chores. Buy a sling before your baby is born! Take him with you (in the sling) when you go to the store and for other errands.
- *Do not use a pacifier.* If your baby sucks fingers, offer your breast. When she starts to cry, let her nurse. If someone gives you a pacifier as a present, throw it away.
- *Take a nap (lie down for 20 minutes) with your baby every day.* Some women have found that this helps them to stay infertile longer.
- *Keep nursing.* When your baby starts eating solids at about six months, she can still nurse. Many babies nurse for a year or two or longer.

Usually, when women nurse like this, they will not have mucus and they will not get a period for about a year.

Now! Some women nurse very often, and they start getting periods again when their baby is five months old. Some women don't get periods for two years or longer. And the way that one baby nurses may be very different from your next one. You have to find your way with each child.

You also have to look for mucus. As long as you are dry and you have no mucus, you are probably not fertile. Once you start to feel wet and see mucus, you have signs that you could ovulate again soon. Of course, if you get a period, that's another sign that you are becoming fertile again. You need to start charting again if you want to know when you are fertile and infertile.

Sometimes, when a mother is away from her baby for an afternoon or more, her milk dries up. If you go away from your baby to work or travel, pumping your milk will help you stay infertile. It will give your baby good nutrition.

No matter how you breastfeed, every mother needs good food and rest. You are eating for two people—and that takes special fuel.

KNOWING YOUR FERTILE AND INFERTILE DAYS WHILE BREASTFEEDING

- Once you notice wet mucus and wet vaginal sensation, start charting your fertility signs again. Charting your waking temperature when you have a baby can be tricky. Do the best you can.
- Look for the Peak Day—your last day of wet mucus or wet vaginal sensation before drying up begins.
- If you have one or two days of wetness, you need *two* days of dry mucus and dry sensation to consider yourself infertile after 6 PM on your second dry day.

  For example, if you are wet on Monday and dry on Tuesday and Wednesday, you can consider yourself infertile after 6 PM on Wednesday. If you are wet on Monday and Tuesday and dry on Wednesday and Thursday, you can consider yourself infertile after 6 PM on Thursday.
- If you have three days or more of wetness, you need *four* days of dry mucus and dry sensation to consider yourself infertile after 6 PM on your fourth dry day after your Peak.

  For example, if you are wet Monday, Tuesday and Wednesday and dry on Thursday, Friday, Saturday and Sunday, you can consider yourself infertile after 6 PM on Sunday.
- If your cervix is soft, open or high (showing that you could be fertile) on a day that your mucus and vaginal sensation tell you that you are *not* fertile, go with what your cervix tells you, and consider yourself fertile.

IF YOU FEED YOUR BABY SOLID FOOD OR WITH A BOTTLE

- The older your baby is, the easier it is to get ovulatory cycles going again.
- Your cycles may come back when you give your baby solid food.
- When you use babysitters or go away from your baby for a day or two, you might ovulate! You can also expect to ovulate when you stop nursing.

Once you see mucus again, it might take several months before you ovulate. Whether they want a new baby or don't feel ready for one, couples often feel frustrated when the woman does not have regular cycles—because they are not sure when the woman is fertile and when she is infertile. You and your husband will need to communicate about your openness to a new pregnancy. You may need to learn how to be intimate in ways other than intercourse.

Some women are very interested in making love when they have small children to care for. Many others feel no interest. Again, the couple needs clear and gentle communication.

Often, when a woman is breastfeeding, her husband will need to be especially gentle with her before and during intercourse. Lovemaking needs to be slow, not quick. Otherwise, intercourse could be very painful for her.

Calling a Fertility Awareness teacher can help you understand your charts.

Some couples who do not feel ready for a new baby use condoms while the woman does not have regular cycles. (See Jane's note about condoms on page 32.)

TO ENCOURAGE OVULATION

A woman may want regular cycles to return so that she can be clearer about when she is fertile and infertile. The couple may not be ready for a new pregnancy. Or, they may feel very open to a new baby.

To encourage regular cycles and ovulation:

- Nurse less frequently.
- If you notice slippery mucus, sleep with a 40-watt bulb on in your bedroom for three nights, then return to darkness. This may help you to ovulate.

If your fertility signs tell you that you have not ovulated yet, try sleeping with light when you notice wet mucus again.

DONNA: After Paul was born, he fell asleep at 8:30 and slept through the night. My mucus came back when Paul was three months old. But my husband (Bill) and I wanted me to stay infertile for at least a year.

I wanted my mucus to dry up so that I would know I was not fertile. We decided that Bill would wake Paul around 11:30 PM, when Bill went to sleep. He put the baby next to me for an extra night nursing. (I usually went to bed before Bill did.) Paul would nurse a bit, and then we went back to sleep. I did not have to get out of bed. At 4:30 AM, he would wake up really hungry, then nurse off and on until 6:30. That extra feeding at 11:30 dried up the mucus almost right away. It did not come back until Paul was 18 months old.

Once I saw the mucus come back, I started charting it again, along with my waking temperature and my cervix. Bill and I were not ready for a new baby yet, so we only made love on days that we knew I was not fertile.

I did not ovulate until Paul was two years old and still nursing some. And I did not get pregnant that cycle.

MARYANNE: I am like most mothers. I have more work to do than I have hours in the day. But I have noticed that if I wait to nurse (so I can finish a chore) until my baby is crying hard, she gets so tense that she can't nurse. I can't relax, either, and then my milk does not let down easily.

My husband and I think that breastmilk is the best nourishment I can give our baby. Nursing helps me space the years between our children and create respectful relationships with them.

So I have realized that my chores can wait. I try my best to nurse on cue—to nurse right when my baby starts to whimper.

SYLVIA: After my son was born, I nursed him about once an hour during the day and two or three times each night. We put his crib (with one side down all the way) right next to our bed so I did not have to move at night to nurse. Still, when he was seven weeks old, I had slippery mucus. That told me I was fertile again and it made me nervous. My husband and I were not ready for a new baby.

Then my son got the flu. I carried him in a sling most of the day so he could rest and I could do my chores. After just a few days, my mucus dried up!

My midwife said that keeping my baby close to me (in the sling) gives my body the message that it has enough to take care of right now. Wearing him in the sling helps my mucus to dry up. And dry mucus tells me that I am not fertile.

My midwife showed me different ways to carry my son in the sling. Depending on the kind of chores I need to do, I can carry him on my back, near my breasts, or on my hip. My midwife knows women who have carried their children in a sling until they are two or three years old.

---

6. Your Menstrual Cycles and Your Health

Your charts tell you when you are fertile and infertile. They also give information about your health. If you find something in your charts that you do not understand, write down your questions. Keep asking them until you get answers that help. Call a Fertility Awareness teacher. Bring your charts and your questions to your doctor or midwife.

If you have a health problem, ask your doctor, "What are my choices?" You may want more than one doctor's opinion. Different people know about different ways to heal. You need to choose what feels right for you and your family. Finding books or a group for people who have your condition can give you more information. If your doctor does not know about a support group for you, start your own!

Here are a few examples of how your charts give information about your health:

OVULATION

Ovulation tells a lot about a woman's health. If a woman does not ovulate regularly (and she is not pregnant, breastfeeding, or near menopause), then she has a sign from her body that she needs to give attention to her health. When a woman does not ovulate regularly, she has a bigger chance of health problems like Poly-Cystic Ovarian Syndrome, diabetes, stroke, and uterine cancer. She may also be infertile.

Doctors often give women birth control pills when they have acne, menstrual cramps, PCOS, mild depression—and when they do not want to get pregnant. The Pill works by stopping the hormones that tell a woman to ovulate. It tells the woman's body to make thick mucus. (Sperm can not live or travel in thick mucus.) The Pill also makes it hard for a fertilized egg to nest in the uterus. Some pills also stop a woman from bleeding. Drug companies say that these pills make a woman's life easier. But these pills carry the same risks of regular birth control pills, and no one has tested what happens when a woman takes them for a long time.

With *Poly-Cystic Ovarian Syndrome (PCOS)*, a woman's eggs get stuck in her ovaries. She does not ovulate regularly. If you have long cycles and lots of split peaks (your mucus gets slippery, but you do not ovulate), you might have PCOS. When a woman has PCOS, she may also be overweight and have hair on her face, high blood pressure, and other problems.

While a woman breastfeeds, it is normal and healthy for her not to ovulate. Women also do not ovulate regularly when they get near menopause. When a woman comes off the Pill, she might not ovulate for several cycles.

If you are not ovulating regularly, then you have a sign from your body to find a healthy diet, to exercise, and to learn how to have a more peaceful mind. Try not eating sugar, soy, products with white flour, or store-bought foods. Try adding eggs, butter, cod liver oil, and a variety of fresh vegetables to your diet. Take an exercise class. Walk more. Spend more time in fresh air with sunlight.

And even if you work hard to change your health, it can take a long time to ovulate regularly. Be gentle with yourself.

DIFFERENT METHODS OF BIRTH CONTROL

Many different kinds of birth control are available. Each kind has advantages and disadvantages. Learn as much as you can about different methods before you choose one. Every couple must decide which method is best for them.

Natural Family Planning (also called Fertility Awareness) helps you understand your menstrual cycle. It does not involve drugs. But if you don't chart correctly or know how to read your charts, you may get a surprise pregnancy.

Condoms do not involve drugs, either. Natural Family Planning and condoms both need the man's cooperation.

The Pill is easy for many couples. Unfortunately, it can cause health problems. If a woman takes the Pill, she has a greater chance of getting breast cancer, blood clots, insulin resistance, and hypothyroidism. She can have less interest in sex. The Pill also takes away some nutrients that a woman needs to have a healthy, smart baby.

If a woman takes the birth control shot Depo-provera, she has a greater chance of bone loss and breast cancer.

Some IUDs give women unnatural hormones.

Some women and men are allergic to spermicide, which is needed when you use a diaphragm or cervical cap.

If you have used a kind of birth control that hurt your cycles, please be gentle with yourself. Many women have returned to healthy cycles by eating well and following the night-lighting techniques described on pages 50-51.

Here is a chart from a woman who did not ovulate during this cycle:

Cycle day	1	2	3	4	5	6	7	8	9	10	11	12	13	14	15	16	17	18	19	20	21	22	23	24	25	26	27	28	29	30	31	32	33	34	35	36	37	38	39	40	41
Intercourse																																									
Temp count																																									

Waking Temperature grid (ranging 97–99°F across cycle days 1–41; temperatures do not jump up and stay up).

Cycle day	1	2	3	4	5	6	7	8	9	10	11	12	13	14	15	16	17	18	19	20	21	22	23	24	25	26	27	28	29	30	31	32	33	34	35	36	37	38	39	40	41
Peak Day							P	1	2	3	4				P	1	2	3				P	1	2	3			P													
Vaginal Sensation																																									
Mucus	mild cramps	light flow	light flow	medium flow	dry	dry	moist, wet	dry	dry	dry	dry	dry	dry	dry	eggwhite	dry	dry	dry	creamy	creamy	itchy	creamy	dry	dry	dry		moist	creamy			new cycle										

She has "false" Peak Days on Days 7, 15, 22, and 28. She never has a true Peak with ovulation. Her temperature does not jump up and stay up during this cycle. There is no place for a coverline. This woman did not ovulate this cycle.

THE THYROID GLAND

The *thyroid gland* is in your neck. It makes hormones that give your body energy and keep a healthy temperature. When you do not make enough thyroid hormones, you feel like you do not have enough energy. When you make too much thyroid hormone, your body feels like it's racing.

Your body gives signs if you might have a thyroid problem. If you have several waking temperatures lower than 97.5, you might have *hypothyroidism*, a slow thyroid. Other signs of hypothyroidism include being overweight, having low energy, cold hands and feet, swollen feet, slow speech, heart palpitations, hair loss, dry or itchy skin, problems with concentrating, muscle aches, shortness of breath, nervousness, constipation, depression, no interest in sex, vaginal infections, painful menstruation, and not ovulating. Because these problems develop slowly and are also signs of stress, your doctor might not check you for hypothyroidism.

With *hyper*thyroidism, you make too much thyroid hormone. You may have high waking temperatures, weight loss, bulging eyes, a fast heart beat, trembling, sweats, problems with sleeping, or infertility.

If you think you have a thyroid problem, your doctor might give you a blood test. There are many ways to read these tests. One doctor might think your test is "normal," while another might think that the same test shows a thyroid problem.

If your temperatures are often lower than 97.5 and you also have some of the problems listed above, find a doctor who reads blood tests for *trends*, not just diseases. If you do have a thyroid problem, please note that doctors often suggest drugs that you could keep taking for years. Naturopaths, homeopaths, and acupuncturists may know natural ways to heal.

People with thyroid problems often have weak *adrenals*. The adrenals may also need treatment for the person's health to improve. Adrenals are glands near your kidneys; they help you when you are under stress.

NIGHT LIGHTING

Before electric lights lit the night sky, many women bled when the moon was new. They ovulated when it was full. Now, most women do not have such regular cycles. They need to chart their fertility signs to know when they are fertile and infertile.

Many women find that sleeping in complete darkness, except for the few days around ovulation, helps their menstrual cycles. This is because our hormones are affected by light. To be healthy, we need sunlight during the day and darkness at night. Some women who do not ovulate regularly or who have difficulty getting pregnant and keeping pregnant have found that night lighting affects their cycles.

Usually, a woman needs to sleep in complete darkness—except around the days she ovulates. Sleeping in complete darkness means that 15 minutes after you turn off your bedroom light, you can not see your hand in front of your face. Getting your room totally dark takes time and attention. You might cover your window one night and the crack under your door the next. While it may take several months, healthier cycles often result.

To get your room totally dark, you can buy "block-out" window blinds. Or, some people cover their windows at night with cardboard from old boxes. You can cover the crack under your door with a towel.

If you need light in the middle of the night (in the bathroom or while nursing), use dim light. You can buy a red bulb (like those used in a photographer's darkroom) from a camera store. Or, cover your lamp with a red scarf.

When you travel, sleep with a folded scarf over your eyes.

To support healthy cycles, sleep in complete darkness. Then:

- After you have two days of wetness, on the night of the second day, sleep with a light on in your room for three nights. Or, keep a light on in a nearby room and keep its door open. After three nights with light, go back to sleeping in darkness for the rest of your cycle.
- If you are not ovulating and have not bled for a month or longer, first sleep in complete darkness for 12 days. Then sleep with a light on for the next three nights. Then go back to sleeping in darkness for two weeks. Continue with this pattern to encourage healthy, ovulatory cycles.
- Once you are pregnant, sleeping in complete darkness can help you keep a healthy pregnancy. After your baby is born, sleep in complete darkness until you are ready to ovulate again.

EMMA I went on the Pill when I was 17 to regulate my cycles, because they were so long and far apart. By the time I was 18 (and still on the Pill), my cramps were very intense on days that I bled. When I was 23, I learned I had endometriosis. For 12 years, I kept taking the Pill. Then I stopped taking it and tried sleeping in darkness except around the days I ovulate. I have been amazed! For five months, I have ovulated within two days of sleeping with light. I feel healthier than I have in years.

---

7. Food for Families

Many people think they save money when they buy the cheapest food they can find. But food is medicine, and so cheap food may actually be very expensive. When we eat food that makes us tired or sick, we can have high medical bills. We might not be able to work or care for our children.

The best way to keep a family healthy is by eating healthy food. Food gives us energy for the day. Children need healthy food to grow strong. Adults need healthy food to keep strong. Diet can also make a difference in a woman's menstrual cycles. In some cultures, young men and women eat special foods for six months before they try to make a baby. When the parents are healthy, their children have a better chance of being healthy.

Unfortunately, the food that is sold in supermarkets and restaurants is often not healthy.

Ask your grandmother what her mother cooked. Before 1940, butter, lard and chicken fat were common. Many people took a spoonful of cod liver oil every day. Corn, canola, and soybean oils were not sold. Crisco and margarine did not exist. People ate much less sugar and ready-made food.

If you want to see whether food makes a difference in your menstrual cycles and your family's health, try an experiment. For a few months, do not eat sugar, soy, or food that contains partially hydrogenated vegetable oil. Do not drink coffee or soda. Find a farmers' market or natural foods store that is near your home. Take a class that teaches how to cook healthy, fresh food.

Some people notice a difference in their health right away when they change their diet. Other people take a long time to notice changes.

UNHEALTHY FOOD

Sugar is also called fructose, corn syrup, sucrose, and dextrose. Eating sugar can make you burn out quickly. It can make you tired. Eating sugar may make some women not ovulate. Sometimes, children who eat sugar get hyper-active. Sugar is in candy, cakes, cookies, cold cereal, ice cream, fruit juices, soft drinks, and canned fruit. Honey and maple syrup can also make you burn out quickly.

White flour. Most bread, pasta, cakes, cookies and pretzels are made with white flour. In the digestive system, white flour works like sugar.

Soy is high in *phyto-estrogens.* Phyto means "from a plant;" estrogen is a hormone that is not healthy when you have too much of it. Soy can cause thyroid problems. It can make it hard for you to absorb calcium, and that can make your bones weak. Margarine, soy cheese, soy milk, soy protein bars, soy protein shakes, soy burgers and tofu are made with soy. Some infant formulas are made with soy. *Miso* (soybean paste) and *tempeh* are okay to eat occasionally because they are fermented. Be sure they're organic.

Milk, eggs, chicken and meat from animals that are raised in factories. When animals are given growth hormones, antibiotics, and grains that have pesticides, these chemicals are passed on to the people who eat their milk and meat.

Caffeine can make it harder for a woman to get pregnant and stay pregnant. It can lower a man's sperm count. Caffeine is in coffee, black tea, soda and chocolate.

Canola, corn, cottonseed, safflower, and soy oils go bad before they are bought; a chemical process makes them smell okay. These oils can destroy cells and DNA and deplete vitamin E. Store-bought salad dressings and mayonnaise are usually made with canola or soy oil. Read labels before you buy!

Trans *fats* are vegetable oils made solid by a chemical process. On food labels, *trans* fats are sometimes called "hydrogenated" or "partially hydrogenated." When men and women eat *trans* fats, they can become infertile. Their babies can be born very small, with many problems. The mother's milk may not be a good quality, which can keep the baby from growing properly. *Trans* fats can cause cancer and heart disease. *Trans* fats are in corn chips and potato chips; bread, cookies and pastries; margarine and vegetable shortening like Crisco; fried foods like donuts, french fries and chicken.

Low-fat foods (like low-fat milk and low-fat yogurt) are not good, because we need fat to digest protein. We need cream to digest the protein in milk.

Farm-raised salmon are usually dyed pink and washed in antibiotics. If the label says "ocean-caught" or "Atlantic" salmon, it can still be farm-raised. *Tuna* and *swordfish* have a lot of mercury. Mercury can make women infertile. The children of women who have mercury in their bodies can have birth defects.

HEALTHY FOOD

Eggs from chickens that graze on organic pastures.

Organic, pastured chicken and beef. These products have necessary minerals and vitamins. Organic lard and pork are also good, and so is liver.

Bone broths and stews made from organic chicken, beef or lamb bones are excellent. (You can buy bones cheaply from butchers and farmers.)

Wild-caught fish that is low in mercury. Wild salmon, sardines canned in olive oil, Alaskan halibut, oysters and stone crab are okay.

Cod liver oil is an excellent source of vitamins A and D. Take a spoonful each day with breakfast, mixed with a little bit of water.

Whole, raw milk from pastured cows. "Raw" means that the milk has not been pasteurized. If a cow gets mostly green grass and hay and if her milk is kept in clean containers, then raw milk is very healthy and safe food. When milk is pasteurized (heated above 118 degrees), the enzymes that we need to digest it start to be destroyed. "Whole" means that the milk has cream in it.

Butter, cheese, and unsweetened yogurt made from raw, organic, whole milk.

Whole grains, beans, nuts and seeds that have been soaked before cooking. Recipes are in *Nourishing Traditions* by Sally Fallon.

Your own salad dressing, made with extra virgin olive oil gives vitamin E.

Fresh fruits that are organic whenever possible and not canned with sugar.

Fresh vegetables (broccoli, spinach, chard, asparagus, green beans, kale, sugar snap peas, dandelion greens, cauliflower, zucchini, beets, turnips, lettuce and cucumbers, for examples) that are organic whenever possible.

Sauerkraut and pickles that were not heated during preparation.

Clean water. If you drink from a well, get your water tested every year!

I know women who ate a lot of food with white flour and *trans* fats (cereal, bread, pasta, pastry, cookies). They ate soy products (soymilk, soyburgers, protein bars, and tofu). They ate potato chips, corn chips, and sugary snacks. They drank coffee, fruit juice and soda. They rarely ate butter or lard, eggs or meat. They rarely ate vegetables. They ate low-fat. And they had problems with their menstrual cycles.

These women wanted healthy cycles, so they tried an experiment. They stopped eating white flour, soy, chips, and sugar. They ate eggs with butter for breakfast. For lunch, they ate cheese, whole grain bread, and salad. They ate beans and brown rice. For dinner, they had beef stew or chicken soup. They bought meat from farmers who let their animals graze on a pasture. With every meal, they ate fresh vegetables and pickles. They took a spoonful of cod liver oil every day. They drank clean water. They stopped drinking fruit juice and soda. Eventually, their cycles got healthier and more regular. Their children and husbands also got healthier.

While you learn to cook in a new way, remember that no diet is right for everyone. Also, from time to time, your nutritional needs can change. Give yourself simple goals. For example, in the first week, you might stop eating desserts every other day. You might start taking a spoonful of cod liver oil. In the second week, cut out all desserts, and find out where you can buy raw milk and fresh vegetables. In the third week, try making yogurt or chicken soup. Here are some menu ideas to get you started:

BREAKFAST
- Eggs cooked in organic lard or organic butter, leftover potatoes, bacon, steamed greens, sauerkraut, a spoonful of cod liver oil.
- Fresh fruit, leftover brown rice with crispy nuts fried in butter, whole yogurt, cod liver oil.
- Porridge, organic raisins and crispy nuts, a piece of leftover organic meat, and cod liver oil.

LUNCH
- Short grain brown rice; beans that were soaked for several hours before cooking; steamed broccoli; a salad with red leaf lettuce, avocados, and cucumbers; dressing made from olive oil and lemon juice; cheese.
- Sardines canned in olive oil, steamed potatoes with butter, dill pickles, steamed chard.

- Whole grain bread; leftover organic chicken in dressing with cider vinegar, garlic and olive oil; cucumber slices; steamed green beans.
- Soup made with chicken broth, fresh spinach (it takes about one minute to cook spinach in broth), and leftover chicken.

SNACKS

- Organic popcorn tossed with coconut oil, organic butter, and celtic salt.
- Crispy nuts (see recipe on page 59).
- Raw cheese made from organic, raw milk.
- Sausage made from organic meats and without MSG or other harmful chemicals.
- Fresh fruit.
- Fresh, organic lemon juice in clean water with a pinch of celtic salt and no sugar.

DINNER

- Organic beef stew, sauerkraut, steamed broccoli.
- Organic roasted chicken, steamed beets tossed in lime juice and olive oil, steamed chard, kale or dandelion greens.
- Wild salmon, baked potato with sour cream, vegetable soup, steamed cauliflower, pickles.
- Organic liver and onions cooked in chicken fat or lard, sauerkraut, steamed green beans.

FEEDING YOUR BABY

Your breastmilk could be the best food you give your baby. But sometimes babies wean when they are young. If your baby stops nursing early, you can make your own formula. Store-bought formula is often made with soy. Soy formula has phyto-estrogens, which are like the hormones in birth control pills. When store-bought formula is made from cows' milk, the cows may have been given antibiotics, growth hormones, or feed grown with pesticides. These chemicals will be in the milk that your children drink. This milk can cause health problems.

Nourishing Traditions by Sally Fallon includes a recipe for making formula with raw milk for babies who wean early.

Once your baby can eat solid food, buy a food grinder so that your baby can eat the food you prepare for your family.

RECIPES

Yogurt
Makes nine cups

½ gallon raw, whole milk
1 cup whole, plain, organic yogurt
   (bought from the store or from the last batch you made)

Heat milk to 110 degrees. (Measure the temperature with a candy thermometer.) Stir in the cup of yogurt. Pour this mixture into a large glass or enamel container. Cover and let sit in a warm place for ten hours, then refrigerate. My oven's pilot light gives just the right amount of heat to make yogurt. I make it after dinner and keep it in the oven at night. Sometimes, I make yogurt with half milk and half cream.

Breakfast Porridge
Serves four

1 cup rolled oats
1 cup warm filtered water
2 tablespoons yogurt, lemon juice or vinegar
1 cup filtered water
½ teaspoon sea salt
1 tablespoon flax seeds (optional)

Mix the oats with warm water and yogurt. Cover and leave overnight in a warm place. In the morning, bring a cup of water with the sea salt to a boil. Add soaked oats. Cover the pot, turn the heat to low, and simmer for 5-10 minutes. Grind the flax seeds. When the oats are cooked, turn off the heat, stir in the flax seeds. Let stand for a few minutes. Serve with butter or cream, crispy nuts, and a bit of honey or maple syrup.

Sauerkraut

Sauerkraut is fermented cabbage that has not been heated. Some people make sauerkraut with cabbage and salt. I make it with cabbage, salt, and whey. Whey is the clear liquid you see that separates from yogurt. Whey helps the cabbage to make enzymes that are good for digestion. My recipe for whey is on the next page.

½ cup of whey (see recipe on page 59)
1 tablespoon unrefined salt *
one small head of organic cabbage (about 1½ pounds), shredded
a large, stainless steel bowl
a meat hammer or pounder   } you can buy these things
a wide-mouth, quart-size glass mason jar   } at a hardware store

Put the shredded cabbage into the stainless steel bowl. Pound it with the meat hammer for about ten minutes. The cabbage will get soft and juice will come out of the cabbage. Cabbage that is very fresh and grown with plenty of water will give the most juice.

Put the whey and the salt into the bowl and toss them with the cabbage and the cabbage juice. Put this mixture into the jar. Push it down with the hammer so that the juice covers the cabbage. Leave one inch between the cabbage and the top of the jar. Cover the jar and let it sit for three days at room temperature. Now the sauerkraut is ready to eat. It will keep in the refrigerator for several months.

Some people like to add caraway seeds to their sauerkraut. Some people add garlic, grated ginger, and a pinch of cayenne pepper.

* Unrefined salt has good minerals. It is grey, beige, or pink—not white. You can find it at a health food store.

Some stores sell special crocks and pickle presses that make it easy to make fermented vegetables like sauerkraut. You can also buy these products from Gold Mine Natural Foods, 800.475.3663; Radiant Life, 888.593.8333; and the Grain and Salt Society, 800.876.7258.

If you want to learn more about making fermented vegetables and other kinds of healthy food, contact the Weston A. Price Foundation (WestonaPrice.org or 202.363.4294). This group has chapters around the world, and many of them offer cooking classes. **Nourishing Traditions** by Sally Fallon and **Wild Fermentation** by Sandor Katz also have excellent recipes for fermented foods.

Whey and Cream Cheese

I know two recipes for making whey and cream cheese. If one of these works for you, great! It's also fun to talk with friends to learn their recipes.

Recipe #1 (Makes about one cup of whey.)
a No. 6 coffee filter cone (purchased in a grocery store)
an unbleached No. 6 coffee filter (purchased in a grocery store)
a glass measuring pitcher that holds two cups of liquid
2 cups of organic yogurt

Put the unbleached coffee filter in the cone. Set the cone with the filter in it on top of the pitcher. Put the yogurt in the filter. Cover it with a loose cloth to keep dust out. Let it sit for about 24 hours. The whey will drip into the pitcher. The cream cheese will be left in the filter. Put the whey in a glass jar. Put the cheese in a glass bowl. Refrigerate them.

Recipe #2 (Makes about two and a half cups of whey)
1 large strainer, set over a bowl
1 clean dish towel
1 quart of organic yogurt
a wooden spoon
a tall pitcher

Set the strainer over a bowl. Line the strainer with the towel. Put the yogurt into the towel. Cover the yogurt with a loose cloth to keep out dust. Let it sit overnight. The whey will drip into the bowl. The milk solids will stay in the towel.

In the morning, make a little sack by tying up the towel with the milk solids inside. Be careful not to squeeze. Tie the sack to a wooden spoon. Place the spoon over a tall pitcher so that more whey can drip out. When the bag stops dripping, the cheese is ready.

The whey will keep in your refrigerator for up to six months. The cream cheese will keep in your refrigerator for about three weeks. Cream cheese is great on toast or baked potatoes. You can mix it with herbs for a dip.

I like to make whey from fil mjolk, a kind of cultured milk that is a little different from yogurt. You can buy a fresh culture of fil mjolk from www.gemcultures.com; or write them at G.E.M Cultures, 30301 Sherwood Road, Fort Bragg, CA 95437-4127.

If your local farmer's market has a cheese-maker, they may sell whey. The Weston Price chapter leader nearest you may also be able to help you make whey or tell you where to buy it.

Chicken Soup
Serves six

1 medium onion, diced
2-3 carrots, cut into 1" pieces
2 stalks celery, cut into ½" pieces
one bunch of parsley, chopped
one parsnip or ½ celery root, cut into bite-sized pieces
2-3 cloves of mashed garlic
4-5 cups of spring water (I use one cup of water for every pound of chicken)
2 teaspoons salt
one 4-5 pound organic, pastured chicken, including the neck and gizzards
  (I prefer a pullet, if I can get one.)

Put everything except the chicken in a soup pot and cover it. Cook over a low flame while you remove the biggest pieces of fat from the chicken. Then, put the chicken into the pot. Cover again and let simmer for an hour and a half. Take the chicken out of the pot. Let it cool for 15 minutes. Take the meat off of the bones and cut it into bite-sized pieces. Put the meat back in the soup.

If you like, add broccoli, brown rice, and/or a can of organic tomatoes.

I know an organic chicken farmer who sells back and neck bones very cheaply. I often make my soup from these bones and find plenty of meat on them. I also buy fish bones and heads (from wild salmon and halibut) quite cheaply at my local supermarket. Sometimes, they give these to me for free and I make fish soup. I use the same recipe I use for the chicken. Again, there's a lot of meat on the fish bones; I remove all the bones before I serve the soup.

Crispy Nuts

4 cups pecan halves
filtered water
2 teaspoons salt

Soak the pecans in filtered water with salt for six hours. Drain them in a strainer or colander. Get all the water out. Spread the nuts in a stainless steel or pyrex baking pan. Bake them at 150 degrees for ten hours or longer, until the nuts are dry and crisp. Store them in a glass jar.

You can also use this recipe with almonds, pumpkin or sunflower seeds.

Crispy nuts make a great snack. You can also put them on hot breakfast cereal, in salads, and on rice.

Vegetable Salad
Serves four

Whisk together:
1 tablespoon unpasteurized cider vinegar or fresh lemon juice
3 tablespoons extra virgin olive oil

1 small cauliflower, cut into bite-sized flowerettes
1 bunch of broccoli, cut into bite-sized flowerettes

Steam the vegetables in a covered pot for about three minutes. Toss them in the dressing. You can also use steamed green beans or steamed beets. This dressing is also good with lettuce and tomatoes.

REBECCA: I was very sick when I got married. I felt too weak to make love. It took four years before I had a baby. After she was born, I felt even more tired. My husband was patient, but my illness was very challenging to our marriage.

Then I decided to learn how to be healthy. I made a commitment to my health and my family's health. My husband and I read Sally Fallon's book, **Nourishing Traditions.** We stopped eating sugar, white flour, vegetable oils and canned vegetables from the store. We started growing our own vegetables and eating salads. We got raw milk from a farmer who does not give his cows hormones or feed with pesticides. Our meat also comes from pastured animals. The food we eat is the way God made it.

When we started this diet, I noticed that I didn't have so many highs and lows. I was also more interested in making love. I've had two more children, and I still have enough energy for the day. Our children get sick sometimes, but they get better after a day or two.

NAOMI: When my husband and I decided to eat a new way for our family's health, I had to change almost everything my mother taught me about preparing food. That was hard. For a year, I didn't visit my relatives much. I had my goal to learn a new way of cooking. I knew that if I talked to other people, I could get confused. I started making soups with bone broths and salads from fresh vegetables. I took away the white bread, cakes and cookies. For snacks, I made popcorn in coconut oil and melted butter on it; I soaked nuts and toasted them. Slowly, my husband, my children, and I got healthier. We have good energy and we sleep well. Once I felt good about the food I served my family, I relaxed around my parents and my friends. It's okay that we cook differently. They see the difference in our health, and sometimes they ask me for recipes.

RACHEL: When my husband and I decided to give our family a healthy diet, we got a Jersey cow for milk and 12 chickens for eggs. We planted a big garden with cabbage, lettuce, broccoli, cucumbers, tomatoes, sweet potatoes, spinach, celery, and melons. My daughters help me can what we grow—enough to take our family through the winter. I store our root vegetables—like beets, potatoes, carrots and onions—in a root cellar. I would love to dig a bigger cellar! I have found that we spend the same amount of money as we did when we bought at the supermarket. Now, we pay for vegetable seeds and to let our cow graze on our neighbor's pasture. We rarely have doctor bills, and our children are learning how to keep a family well fed and healthy.

8. Books and Other Resources

Many people learn how to keep their families healthy by reading books. With everything that you read, you have to decide which ideas are right for your family—and which ones are not right.

Your midwife and your library have books that you can borrow for free.

A librarian can also help you find information about health problems. For example, if your doctor says that you need a hysterectomy, ask a librarian to help you find a book or search on a computer for information about other choices. If you have a child who is autistic or mentally retarded, a librarian can help you find books or groups with helpful information.

Many people like to own their favorite books. If you have books about herbs and homeopathy, one of them might have a remedy for menstrual cramps that works for you or your daughters. You can buy books at half price from used book stores. Look in the yellow pages under "Books," then look for "Used Books."

I think every family should have a dictionary.

Your best book might be the one you write yourself. Buy a notebook and keep a record of the remedies that help when someone in your family has a toothache, diarrhea, or a yeast infection. Give each condition a whole page so you can find your notes easily when you need them.

You can also write down questions in your notebook. When you visit your doctor or meet with a Natural Family Planning teacher, bring your notebook.

Here are some books that I find helpful:

Family Planning
The Garden of Fertility by Katie Singer. In this book, I describe more about charting than I do here. www.GardenofFertility.com has blank charts and sells a study guide for people who want to teach Fertility Awareness.

CycleBeads help women know which days they can get pregnant, and which days conception would probably not happen. CycleBeads look like a necklace with two colors. They can only be used by women whose cycles are regularly 26-32 days long. It takes about 20 minutes to learn how to use CycleBeads. They are about 95% effective when used correctly. For more information, contact The Institute for Reproductive Health of Georgetown University, 4301 Connecticut Av. NW, #310, Washington, DC 20008; 202.687.1392; www.irh.org; www.cyclebeads.com.

Food
Nourishing Traditions by Sally Fallon. Explains why people need animal fats like butter and lard from organic, grass-fed livestock; sauerkraut; and raw dairy. It includes over 700 recipes and a chapter on feeding babies. Order from Radiant Life, www.RadiantLife.org or call 888.593.8333.

Wise Traditions in Food, Farming & the Healing Arts. A magazine with articles about good food and health care. Order from the Weston A. Price Foundation, PMB #106-380, 4200 Wisconsin Avenue, NW, Washington DC 20016. 202.363.4394; www.westonaprice.org

Herbs
Herbal Healing for Women by Rosemary Gladstar. Explains how to make herbal teas, salves, pills, and tinctures for menstrual cramps, skin problems, endometriosis, vaginal infections, pregnancy, and menopause.

The New Menopausal Years the Wise Woman Way: Alternative Approaches for Women 30 to 90 by Susun Weed. Gives remedies for cramps, thyroid problems, vaginal dryness, yeast infections, hot flashes, etc.; www.susunweed.com

Wise Woman Herbal for the Childbearing Year by Susun Weed. A wonderful book for pregnant women.

Pregnancy, Breastfeeding, & Early Childhood
Breastfeeding Your Baby, Revised, by Sheila Kitzinger. Gives advice for all kinds of breastfeeding problems.

The Family Bed, by Tine Thevinin. Describes how sleeping together can help parents and children to sleep better and feel more secure.

Homeopathy for Pregnancy, Birth & Your Baby's First Year by Miranda Castro.

A Kid's Herb Book by Lesley Tierra. Explains differences between herbs and weeds; gives recipes for making vinegar, compost, and simple medicinal teas.

Mothering. A magazine with stories about breastfeeding, the family bed, diapers, autism, vaccines, encouraging creativity, etc. Mothering believes that children have needs and rights and it recognizes parents as experts. The magazine has ads from companies that sell baby slings. www.mothering.org; 800-984-8116.

Helpful People
The Fertility Awareness Network, based in New York, can help you find a teacher to make sure you understand your charts. www.fertaware.com/fan_resources.html; 212.475.4490.

The Couple to Couple League, based in Ohio, teaches Natural Family Planning with a Catholic perspective. www.ccli.org; 513.471.2000.

La Leche League is a group of volunteers around the world who give support and advice to breastfeeding mothers. www.LaLecheLeague.org; 847-519-7730.

The Weston A. Price Foundation has chapter leaders who can help you locate organic food and raw dairy products in your area. Some chapters offer cooking classes. www.WestonAPrice.org; 202.363.4394.

Ask your midwife where you can buy a sling. Buy one before your baby arrives!

9. Testing How Well You Know Natural Family Planning

This test can help you find out what you know and don't know about Natural Family Planning before you start using it to space your children. You and your husband can each take the test. Go over your answers together. If you are not sure about an answer, call a teacher. You can find teachers by calling The Fertility Awareness Network at 212.475.4490 or The Couple to Couple League at 513.471.2000.

1. What is Natural Family Planning?

It is a natural system for couples to know when the woman is fertile and not fertile by charting her waking temperature and her cervical mucus. This system is also called Fertility Awareness.

2. What is the difference between a "menstrual cycle" and a "menstrual period?"

A cycle starts on the first day of menstrual bleeding, and it ends the day before you start bleeding again. The days when you bleed are your period.

3. What is the first day of your cycle?

The day you start bleeding.

4. Name two things that mucus can do to help you get pregnant.
a. Mucus can keep sperm alive for up to five days.
b. It helps sperm travel from your cervix to a fallopian tube at ovulation.

5. How long does a ripe egg live at ovulation?
12–24 hours

6. A woman can ovulate more than once in a menstrual cycle. True or False
False. Even when two eggs are released (starting twins that do not look alike), it's still only one ovulation.

7. How do you know if you are fertile or infertile while you're bleeding?
While you bleed, you can not tell if you have mucus. During the first 12 cycles that you chart, consider yourself fertile while you bleed and spot.

Once you have had 12 cycles that are all 26 days or longer, you can consider yourself infertile during the first five days of your cycle.

If one of your last 12 cycles was shorter than 26 days, you are infertile during your cycle's first three days.

8. How and when do you check for mucus?
At least three times a day, before urinating, wash your hands and take a mucus sample from just inside the vagina. Wash your hands and take your sample with your finger or with a toilet tissue. You want to know if your sample is dry, tacky, creamy, or stretchy like eggwhite.

9. When charting your mucus, what do you write down?
The wettest sample that you had during the day.

10. What is vaginal sensation? How do you check for it?
Vaginal sensation is the feeling of being wet or dry. During the day, you notice what you feel. When you wipe yourself with tissue after urinating, you can also notice if the lips of your vagina feel dry or wet.

11. When charting your vaginal sensation, what do you write down?
"*D*" if your vaginal sensation always felt dry.
"*W*" if it ever felt wet during the day.

12. After your period, you have a wet sensation on your vaginal lips, but no mucus. Do you consider yourself fertile or infertile?
Fertile.

13. What is the Peak Day?
The *last* day of wet vaginal sensation or slippery mucus before your mucus starts to dry up. Your Peak Day is often the day that you ovulate.

14. Can you have more than one Peak Day in a cycle? Explain.
Yes. Your mucus can be wet, then dry up for a day or more even though you have not ovulated. This is called a false Peak. You can have several false Peaks before you have a true Peak. You have a true Peak when your mucus dries up *and* your temperatures get high and stay high: you can confirm that you ovulated.

15. What is arousal fluid and how is it different from mucus?
Arousal fluid makes a woman's vagina slippery when she wants sex so that intercourse will not be painful for her. Arousal fluid can not keep sperm alive. Mucus can also be slippery; and mucus can keep sperm alive for up to five days.

16. How can you tell whether you are wet from arousal fluid or mucus?
You check for mucus three times each day.

17. Which hormone is strongest before you ovulate? What does this hormone do?
Estrogen. While your eggs grow in their shells, they make estrogen. Every cycle, estrogen builds a new layer of blood in your uterus. It tells your cervix to make mucus. It makes your temperature cool.

18. Which hormone is strong *after* ovulation? What does this hormone do?
Progesterone. The empty egg shell makes progesterone after ovulation. Progestrone dries your mucus and makes your body temperature warm.

19. Name three reasons to chart your waking temperature every day.

1. It can tell you that you have ovulated.
2. If you have several temperatures below 97.5, you have a sign that you might have a thyroid problem.
3. It can tell you that you are pregnant.

20. Which activities could change your waking temperature?

Just before taking it, you make love, eat or drink, climb stairs, have a bowel movement, sleep on a heated waterbed or with an electric blanket, don't get enough sleep, or you drink alcohol the night before. Being sick or taking your temperature later or earlier than usual can also affect it.

21. Before ovulation, your waking temperature tells you when you are fertile or infertile. True or False

False. Before ovulation, your temperature can NOT tell you whether or not you are fertile.

22. After your period and before ovulation, how do you know if you are fertile?

By charting your vaginal sensation and mucus.

If you have been dry all day, you are considered infertile after 6 PM. The next day, you need to be dry all day again to consider yourself infertile that evening.

Once you have mucus or a wet sensation, you are fertile until you confirm that you ovulated.

Also, if your cervix is soft, high in the vaginal canal, or open, consider yourself fertile.

If you are breastfeeding, you will need the special rules on page 44.

23. Using the rules for mucus, how do you know that you have ovulated and are no longer fertile for that cycle?

a. Locate your Peak Day
b. Count four days in a row of mucus and vaginal sensation that are dryer than they were on the Peak Day.
c. After 6 PM on the fourth day in a row of mucus that is dryer than the Peak Day's mucus, your egg is gone and you are infertile for the rest of that cycle.

24. Using the waking temperature, how can you tell that you have ovulated and you are infertile?

a. When your temperature goes up, count back six temperatures, starting with the first low temperature before it jumps up.

b. Draw a coverline one tenth of a degree above the highest of the six low temperatures.

c. You need three days of temperatures in a row above the coverline. After 6 PM of the 3rd evening above the line, your egg is gone. You are infertile for the rest of that cycle.

25. Sticky mucus before ovulation is a sign that you are fertile. After ovulation, the same kind of mucus can be a sign that you are not fertile. True or False?

True. Once you have had four days of mucus that are dryer than your Peak Day mucus, you are infertile after 6 PM of that fourth day. So if your Peak Day mucus was slippery like eggwhite, then four days of sticky mucus (which is dryer than eggwhite) after your Peak Day would mean you are infertile for the rest of that cycle.

26. How can you tell by your chart that you are pregnant?

When you have 18 days of high temperatures above your coverline, you are probably pregnant.

27. What are the best days to have intercourse if you want to get pregnant and your husband has a normal sperm count?

When you notice slippery mucus and wet vaginal sensation, have intercourse once each day.

28. What are the best days to have intercourse if you want to get pregnant and your husband has a low sperm count?

When you notice slippery mucus and wet vaginal sensation, have intercourse every other day.

29. What happens during an anovulatory cycle?

The woman does not ovulate. This is common when the woman is coming off the Pill, breastfeeding or weaning, near menopause, and when she has Poly-Cystic Ovarian Syndrome (PCOS). Anovulatory cycles are also common with teenagers.

30. What is Poly-Cystic Ovarian Syndrome (PCOS)?

When a woman has PCOS, her eggs get stuck in her ovaries. She has problems ovulating. She may have very long cycles. She may be overweight. She may also have hair on her face, high blood pressure, and other problems.

31. What does an anovulatory chart look like?

The mucus is usually dry or sticky; it does not get slippery. Also, the temperature might go up, but it does not stay up.

32. How can charts help you know whether you might have ovarian cysts?

If you have a false Peak more than once a year. A false Peak is when your mucus gets wet and then dries up—but your temperature does not go up. A false Peak is a sign that your eggs are growing—but you are not ovulating.

33. How can you tell if you have miscarried?

You have had 18 days of temperatures above your coverline (telling you that you are pregnant), and then you start bleeding.

34. What is hypothyroidism? How do charts tell whether you might have it?

People with hypothyroidism have a thyroid that works slowly. The thyroid is in charge of your temperature and your energy. Waking temperatures below 97.5 can mean that you may have this condition. Other symptoms include: cold hands and feet, depression, and being overweight. A person with thyroid problems may also need to make their adrenal glands stronger.

35. Name four dietary changes that could help your menstrual cycles.

1. Stop eating sugar, including fruit juice, cookies, cakes, jam, and honey.
2. Stop eating soy products, including soy protein bars, soymilk, margarine, and tofu.
3. Buy organic, fresh food whenever possible, and start cooking!
4. Take a teaspoon of cod liver oil every day.

36. Name seven things new mothers can do to help them be infertile for a year or two or more—and space their children.

1. In the baby's first few months, nurse once or twice every hour.
2. Nurse several times at night.
3. Keep nursing, even when your baby starts to eat solid food.
4. Wear your baby in a sling during the day.
5. Don't use pacifiers.
6. Sleep in darkness.
7. Take a nap with your baby for 20 minutes every day.

37. How does a breastfeeding mother know that she is not fertile?
Her mucus and vaginal sensation are dry.

38. How does a breastfeeding mother know that her fertility is coming back?
She starts to notice wet mucus and wet vaginal sensation again.

39. If you have questions about your charts, where can you find a Fertility Awareness teacher?
Call the Fertility Awareness Network, 212.475.4490. The Couple to Couple League offers classes with a Catholic orientation at 513.471.2000. Also, the Billings Ovulation Method Association teaches about mucus (not temperature) with a Catholic orientation. Their number is 651.699.8139.

QUESTIONS ONLY YOU & YOUR HUSBAND CAN ANSWER
40. Most women are fertile for one third to one half of their cycle. If you want to make love while you are fertile and you don't want to get pregnant, what are your choices?

41. If you have a hard time getting pregnant, what medical treatments do you think are okay?

42. When should people learn Natural Family Planning?

FOR EACH OF THE FOLLOWING CHARTS:

- When is she infertile? When is she fertile?
- Which is the Peak Day?
- Where is the coverline?
- When does she know that her egg is gone for this cycle and that she is infertile?
- If she wants to get pregnant, when are the best days to try?
- Does her chart say anything about her health that she should talk about with her doctor?

Days this cycle _____

Cycle day	1	2	3	4	5	6	7	8	9	10	11	12	13	14	15	16	17	18	19	20	21	22	23	24	25	26	27	28	29	30	31	32	33	34	35	36	37	38	39	40	41
Intercourse																																									
Temp count																																									

Waking Temperature (chart grid with plotted temperatures)

Cycle day	1	2	3	4	5	6	7	8	9	10	11	12	13	14	15	16	17	18	19	20	21	22	23	24	25	26	27	28	29	30	31	32	33	34	35	36	37	38	39	40	41
Peak Day																																									
Vaginal Sensation						D	D	W	W	W	W	W	W	W	W	W	W	D	D	D	D	D	D	D	D	D	D	D	D	D	D										
Mucus	heavy flow	heavy flow	med. heavy flow	light flow	spotting	spotting	dry	dry	slight cream	milky	milky - bouncy	milky - bouncy	creamy	creamy	slight stretch	strechy	dry	dry	dry	dry	dry	dry	dry	dry	dry	dry	dry	dry	slightly creamy	dry	dry	new cycle									

This cycle is 31 days long. Sarah is infertile after 6 PM on Days 7 and 8. Her fertile time starts on Day 9. Her Peak Day is Day 16. Her coverline is at 98.0. Her mucus and her temperature tell her that her egg for this cycle is gone and that she is infertile again at 6 PM on Day 20. If she and her husband have intercourse during this cycle after 6PM on Day 20, she will not get pregnant. If they want a new pregnancy, their best days to try are Days 14, 15, and 16.

Days this cycle _____

Cycle day	1	2	3	4	5	6	7	8	9	10	11	12	13	14	15	16	17	18	19	20	21	22	23	24	25	26	27	28	29	30	31	32	33	34	35	36	37	38	39	40	41
Intercourse																																									
Temp count																																									
Waking Temperature																																									
Cycle day	1	2	3	4	5	6	7	8	9	10	11	12	13	14	15	16	17	18	19	20	21	22	23	24	25	26	27	28	29	30	31	32	33	34	35	36	37	38	39	40	41
Peak Day																																									
Vaginal Sensation																																									
Mucus	mild cramps	light flow	light flow	medium flow	dry	dry	moist, wet	dry	dry	dry	dry	dry	dry	eggwhite	dry	dry	dry	creamy	creamy	itchy	creamy	dry	dry	dry	moist	creamy					new cycle										

This cycle is 30 days long. Gabrielle is infertile after 6 PM Days 5 and 6. Day 7 is a false Peak Day. Because she has four dry days after this Peak Day, she is infertile after 6 PM on Day 11. Because her temperature does not go up and stay up around Day 7, she knows that she did not ovulate. She is also infertile after 6 PM on Days 12, 13 and 14. Day 15 is another false Peak Day.

She has mucus on Day 19 that is wetter than it was on the days before—so she should consider herself possibly fertile starting on Day 19. Day 22 is another false Peak Day. Because she did not check her mucus on Day 26, she should think that she is possibly fertile that evening. There is no place for a coverline in this cycle, because her temperature does not go up and stay up.

In this cycle, Gabrielle did not ovulate. If she is not breastfeeding and she continues not to ovulate, she might talk with her doctor to see if she has PCOS. Also, eight of her temperatures are below 97.5. She might have hypothyroidism.

		# Days this cycle _____

Cycle day	1 2 3 4 5 6 7 8 9 10 11 12 13 14 15 16 17 18 19 20 21 22 23 24 25 26 27 28 29 30 31 32 33 34 35 36 37 38 39 40 41
Intercourse	
Temp count	

Waking Temperature chart — temperatures recorded in columns, with scale from 96.9 up through 97 and 98 to 99 for each cycle day.

Cycle day	1 2 3 4 5 6 7 8 9 10 11 12 13 14 15 16 17 18 19 20 21 22 23 24 25 26 27 28 29 30 31 32 33 34 35 36 37 38 39 40 41
Peak Day	
Vaginal Sensation	

Mucus (by cycle day):
1. light flow
2. heavy flow
3. medium – heavy
4. medium – light
5. light flow
6. spotting
7. dry
8. dry
9. dry
10. dry
11. dry
12. dry
13. moist
14. wet
15. wet
16. wet – creamy
17. moist
18. wet
19. eggwhite
20. eggwhite, 1 1/2"
21. dry
22. dry
23. creamy
24. eggwhite, 1"
25. wet
26. wet
27. dry
28. dry
29. dry
30. dry, drank wine
31. yeast infection
32. yeast infection
33. dry
34. itchy
35. dry
36. dry
37. dry
38. new cycle

This cycle is 38 days long. Stephanie is infertile after 6 PM on Days 7, 8, 9, 10, 11 and 12. Her fertile time starts on Day 13. She has a false Peak Day on Day 20. Her true Peak Day is Day 26. By her mucus, she knows that her egg is gone and she is infertile starting on Day 30 after 6 PM. Her coverline is at 97.1. By her temperature, she is infertile on Day 27, after 6 PM. Her mucus tells her to wait longer to consider herself infertile. She should wait until after 6 PM on Day 30 to consider herself infertile. To get pregnant, she might think that Days 18, 19, 20 and 23 are the best days for her and her husband to try, because she felt wet and saw mucus on those days. But their best day to try is Day 24, the last day of eggwhite before her temperature goes up.

Stephanie's low temperatures show that she may have hypothyroidism.

Cycle day	1	2	3	4	5	6	7	8	9	10	11	12	13	14	15	16	17	18	19	20	21	22	23	24	25	26	27	28	29	30	31	32	33	34	35	36	37	38	39	40	41
Intercourse																																									
Temp count																																									

Waking Temperature (plotted chart, values 99 down to 97 9, with circled/plotted temperatures)

Cycle day	1	2	3	4	5	6	7	8	9	10	11	12	13	14	15	16	17	18	19	20	21	22	23	24	25	26	27	28	29	30	31	32	33	34	35	36	37	38	39	40	41
Peak Day																																									
Vaginal Sensation				D	D	D	W	W	W	D	D	D	D	D	D	D	D	D	D	D	D	D																			

Mucus:
- Day 1: light flow
- Day 2: light flow
- Day 3: light
- Day 4: light
- Day 5: spotting
- Day 6: dry
- Day 7: dry
- Day 8: dry
- Day 9: creamy
- Day 10: eggwhite
- Day 11: eggwhite
- Day 12: dry
- Day 13: dry
- Day 14: dry
- Day 26: new cycle

This cycle is 25 days long. Elsa is infertile after 6 PM on Days 6, 7 and 8. Her fertile time starts on Day 9. Her Peak Day is Day 11. Her coverline is at 97.7. By her mucus, she knows that her egg is gone and she is infertile after 6 PM on Day 15. By her temperature, she knows that her egg is gone and she is infertile after 6 PM on Day 14. Her mucus tells her to wait longer to consider herself infertile. She should wait until after 6 PM on Day 15 to consider herself infertile.

Because this cycle is short (only 25 days long), she can consider only the first three days of her period infertile for her next 12 cycles.

To get pregnant, her best days to try are Days 9, 10, and 11.

Elsa has eight temperatures below 97.5; she might have hypothyroidism.

Cycle day	1	2	3	4	5	6	7	8	9	10	11	12	13	14	15	16	17	18	19	20	21	22	23	24	25	26	27	28	29	30	31	32	33	34	35	36	37	38	39	40	41
Intercourse		✓							✓										✓				✓																		
Temp count																																									

Waking Temperature (chart grid, degrees 97–99)

Cycle day	1	2	3	4	5	6	7	8	9	10	11	12	13	14	15	16	17	18	19	20	21	22	23	24	25	26	27	28	29	30	31	32	33	34	35	36	37	38	39	40	41
Peak Day																																									
Vaginal Sensation																																									
Mucus	light flow	light flow	very light		dry	dry	rubbery & crumbly	yellow, sticky	wet, eggwhite	eggwhite, 6"	less, still clear	scant, same	dry	dry	dry	dry	dry	dry	dry																						

Linda can not consider herself infertile on Days 4 and 5 because she did not chart on those days. She is infertile after 6 PM on Days 6 and 7. Her fertile phase starts on Day 8. Her Peak Day is Day 13. Her coverline is at 97.8. By her mucus, she knows that her egg is gone and she is infertile after 6 PM on Day 17. By her temperature, she knows that her egg is gone and she is infertile after 6 PM on Day 16. Her mucus tells her to wait longer to consider herself infertile. She should wait until after 6 PM on Day 17 to consider herself infertile.

To get pregnant, her best days to try are Days 10, 11, 12, and 13.

Linda and her husband were not trying to get pregnant this cycle. However, they had intercourse on Day 9, a fertile day. She knew she was pregnant on Day 30, when she had 18 temperatures above her coverline.

A SUMMARY OF RULES FOR NOT GETTING PREGNANT

During the Menstrual Period

Because you can have mucus while you bleed or spot (and not be able to see or feel it), consider your period a fertile time during your first 12 charted cycles. Once you have had 12 ovulatory cycles in a row that are each 26 days or longer, you can consider yourself infertile Days 1 through 5. If you have had a cycle that is 25 days or shorter, you can consider yourself infertile Days 1 through 3.

Dry Day Rule

In a dry vagina, sperm can not live more than four hours. Once you notice mucus or wet vaginal sensation, you are fertile. Intercourse can lead to pregnancy. After the period (*and before ovulation*), you are infertile after 6 PM if you have been dry all day. The next day, you need to be dry all day again to call yourself infertile after 6 PM.

Peak Day Rule

The last day of wet mucus or wet vaginal sensation is called the Peak Day. Women usually ovulate on the Peak Day. When your mucus has dried up for several days, you have a sign from your body that your egg is gone for this cycle. You are infertile after 6 PM when you have four days in a row of mucus and vaginal sensation that are drier than your Peak Day.

Temperature Shift Rule

When your temperature goes up, count back six low temperatures; draw a coverline one tenth of a degree above the highest of these low temperatures. When your temperature is above your coverline for three days in a row, you are infertile after 6 PM on that third day.

If You Are Not Sure Whether You Are Fertile or Infertile

If you do not want a new pregnancy and you are not sure whether you are fertile or infertile, do not have intercourse. Consider yourself fertile until all of your signs tell you that you are infertile. If your mucus and temperature do not match, listen to the one that tells you that you are still fertile.

A SUMMARY OF WAYS TO HELP YOU GET PREGNANT

1. If your husband's sperm count is normal, have intercourse each day you have wet mucus or wet vaginal sensation. If his sperm count is low, have intercourse every other day that you have wetness. Either way, try to have intercourse on your Peak Day.

2. Try to make love on the first morning that your temperature jumps up.

3. Eat a healthy diet. Exercise regularly. Sleep in total darkness except around the days you have slippery mucus. (Read more about night lighting on pages 50-51.)

Fertility Cycle #_____

Start Date _____   # Days this cycle _____

Cycle day	1	2	3	4	5	6	7	8	9	10	11	12	13	14	15	16	17	18	19	20	21	22	23	24	25	26	27	28	29	30	31	32	33	34	35	36	37	38	39	40	41
Date																																									
Intercourse																																									
Time Temp Taken																																									
Temp count																																									

Waking Temperature (grid ranging from 99 down to 96.9 degrees)

Cycle day	1	2	3	4	5	6	7	8	9	10	11	12	13	14	15	16	17	18	19	20	21	22	23	24	25	26	27	28	29	30	31	32	33	34	35	36	37	38	39	40	41
Peak Day																																									
Vaginal Sensation																																									
Cervix (● o O / F M S)																																									
Mucus						BSE																																			

Cycle day	1	2	3	4	5	6	7	8	9	10	11	12	13	14	15	16	17	18	19	20	21	22	23	24	25	26	27	28	29	30	31	32	33	34	35	36	37	38	39	40	41
Miscellaneous:																																									

A SUMMARY OF RULES FOR NOT GETTING PREGNANT

During the Menstrual Period

Because you can have mucus while you bleed or spot (and not be able to see or feel it), consider your period a fertile time during your first 12 charted cycles. Once you have had 12 ovulatory cycles in a row that are each 26 days or longer, you can consider yourself infertile Days 1 through 5. If you have had a cycle that is 25 days or shorter, you can consider yourself infertile Days 1 through 3.

Dry Day Rule

In a dry vagina, sperm can not live more than four hours. Once you notice mucus or wet vaginal sensation, you are fertile. Intercourse can lead to pregnancy. After the period (*and before ovulation*), you are infertile after 6 PM if you have been dry all day. The next day, you need to be dry all day again to call yourself infertile after 6 PM.

Peak Day Rule

The last day of wet mucus or wet vaginal sensation is called the Peak Day. Women usually ovulate on the Peak Day. When your mucus has dried up for several days, you have a sign from your body that your egg is gone for this cycle. You are infertile after 6 PM when you have four days in a row of mucus and vaginal sensation that are drier than your Peak Day.

Temperature Shift Rule

When your temperature goes up, count back six low temperatures; draw a coverline one tenth of a degree above the highest of these low temperatures. When your temperature is above your coverline for three days in a row, you are infertile after 6 PM on that third day.

If You Are Not Sure Whether You Are Fertile or Infertile

If you do not want a new pregnancy and you are not sure whether you are fertile or infertile, do not have intercourse. Consider yourself fertile until all of your signs tell you that you are infertile. If your mucus and temperature do not match, listen to the one that tells you that you are still fertile.

A SUMMARY OF WAYS TO HELP YOU GET PREGNANT

1. If your husband's sperm count is normal, have intercourse each day you have wet mucus or wet vaginal sensation. If his sperm count is low, have intercourse every other day that you have wetness. Either way, try to have intercourse on your Peak Day.

2. Try to make love on the first morning that your temperature jumps up.

3. Eat a healthy diet. Exercise regularly. Sleep in total darkness except around the days you have slippery mucus. (Read more about night lighting on pages 50-51.)

Fertility Cycle #_____

Start Date _____   # Days this cycle _____

Cycle day	1	2	3	4	5	6	7	8	9	10	11	12	13	14	15	16	17	18	19	20	21	22	23	24	25	26	27	28	29	30	31	32	33	34	35	36	37	38	39	40	41
Date																																									
Intercourse																																									
Time Temp Taken																																									
Temp count																																									

Waking Temperature — grid of temperature values (99, 98, 97, 96) with decimal rows 9 through 1 for each whole degree, repeated across cycle days 1–41.

Cycle day	1	2	3	4	5	6	7	8	9	10	11	12	13	14	15	16	17	18	19	20	21	22	23	24	25	26	27	28	29	30	31	32	33	34	35	36	37	38	39	40	41
Peak Day																																									
Vaginal Sensation																																									

Cervix: ● o O / F M S

Mucus — (blank grid; BSE noted at cycle day 7)

Cycle day	1	2	3	4	5	6	7	8	9	10	11	12	13	14	15	16	17	18	19	20	21	22	23	24	25	26	27	28	29	30	31	32	33	34	35	36	37	38	39	40	41
Miscellaneous:																																									

A SUMMARY OF RULES FOR NOT GETTING PREGNANT

During the Menstrual Period

Because you can have mucus while you bleed or spot (and not be able to see or feel it), consider your period a fertile time during your first 12 charted cycles. Once you have had 12 ovulatory cycles in a row that are each 26 days or longer, you can consider yourself infertile Days 1 through 5. If you have had a cycle that is 25 days or shorter, you can consider yourself infertile Days 1 through 3.

Dry Day Rule

In a dry vagina, sperm can not live more than four hours. Once you notice mucus or wet vaginal sensation, you are fertile. Intercourse can lead to pregnancy. After the period (*and before ovulation*), you are infertile after 6 PM if you have been dry all day. The next day, you need to be dry all day again to call yourself infertile after 6 PM.

Peak Day Rule

The last day of wet mucus or wet vaginal sensation is called the Peak Day. Women usually ovulate on the Peak Day. When your mucus has dried up for several days, you have a sign from your body that your egg is gone for this cycle. You are infertile after 6 PM when you have four days in a row of mucus and vaginal sensation that are drier than your Peak Day.

Temperature Shift Rule

When your temperature goes up, count back six low temperatures; draw a coverline one tenth of a degree above the highest of these low temperatures. When your temperature is above your coverline for three days in a row, you are infertile after 6 PM on that third day.

If You Are Not Sure Whether You Are Fertile or Infertile

If you do not want a new pregnancy and you are not sure whether you are fertile or infertile, do not have intercourse. Consider yourself fertile until all of your signs tell you that you are infertile. If your mucus and temperature do not match, listen to the one that tells you that you are still fertile.

A SUMMARY OF WAYS TO HELP YOU GET PREGNANT

1. If your husband's sperm count is normal, have intercourse each day you have wet mucus or wet vaginal sensation. If his sperm count is low, have intercourse every other day that you have wetness. Either way, try to have intercourse on your Peak Day.

2. Try to make love on the first morning that your temperature jumps up.

3. Eat a healthy diet. Exercise regularly. Sleep in total darkness except around the days you have slippery mucus. (Read more about night lighting on pages 50-51.)

Fertility Cycle #_____

Start Date _____   # Days this cycle _____

Cycle day	1	2	3	4	5	6	7	8	9	10	11	12	13	14	15	16	17	18	19	20	21	22	23	24	25	26	27	28	29	30	31	32	33	34	35	36	37	38	39	40	41
Date																																									
Intercourse																																									
Time Temp Taken																																									
Temp count																																									

Waking Temperature (scale: 99, 9–1, 98, 9–1, 97, 9–1, 96, 9 repeated for each cycle day)

Cycle day	1	2	3	4	5	6	7	8	9	10	11	12	13	14	15	16	17	18	19	20	21	22	23	24	25	26	27	28	29	30	31	32	33	34	35	36	37	38	39	40	41
Peak Day																																									
Vaginal Sensation																																									
Cervix (● o O / F M S)																																									
Mucus						BSE																																			

Cycle day	1	2	3	4	5	6	7	8	9	10	11	12	13	14	15	16	17	18	19	20	21	22	23	24	25	26	27	28	29	30	31	32	33	34	35	36	37	38	39	40	41
Miscellaneous:																																									

A SUMMARY OF RULES FOR NOT GETTING PREGNANT

During the Menstrual Period

Because you can have mucus while you bleed or spot (and not be able to see or feel it), consider your period a fertile time during your first 12 charted cycles. Once you have had 12 ovulatory cycles in a row that are each 26 days or longer, you can consider yourself infertile Days 1 through 5. If you have had a cycle that is 25 days or shorter, you can consider yourself infertile Days 1 through 3.

Dry Day Rule

In a dry vagina, sperm can not live more than four hours. Once you notice mucus or wet vaginal sensation, you are fertile. Intercourse can lead to pregnancy. After the period (*and before ovulation*), you are infertile after 6 PM if you have been dry all day. The next day, you need to be dry all day again to call yourself infertile after 6 PM.

Peak Day Rule

The last day of wet mucus or wet vaginal sensation is called the Peak Day. Women usually ovulate on the Peak Day. When your mucus has dried up for several days, you have a sign from your body that your egg is gone for this cycle. You are infertile after 6 PM when you have four days in a row of mucus and vaginal sensation that are drier than your Peak Day.

Temperature Shift Rule

When your temperature goes up, count back six low temperatures; draw a coverline one tenth of a degree above the highest of these low temperatures. When your temperature is above your coverline for three days in a row, you are infertile after 6 PM on that third day.

If You Are Not Sure Whether You Are Fertile or Infertile

If you do not want a new pregnancy and you are not sure whether you are fertile or infertile, do not have intercourse. Consider yourself fertile until all of your signs tell you that you are infertile. If your mucus and temperature do not match, listen to the one that tells you that you are still fertile.

A SUMMARY OF WAYS TO HELP YOU GET PREGNANT

1. If your husband's sperm count is normal, have intercourse each day you have wet mucus or wet vaginal sensation. If his sperm count is low, have intercourse every other day that you have wetness. Either way, try to have intercourse on your Peak Day.

2. Try to make love on the first morning that your temperature jumps up.

3. Eat a healthy diet. Exercise regularly. Sleep in total darkness except around the days you have slippery mucus. (Read more about night lighting on pages 50-51.)

Fertility Cycle # _____

Start Date _____   # Days this cycle _____

Cycle day	1	2	3	4	5	6	7	8	9	10	11	12	13	14	15	16	17	18	19	20	21	22	23	24	25	26	27	28	29	30	31	32	33	34	35	36	37	38	39	40	41
Date																																									
Intercourse																																									
Time Temp Taken																																									
Temp count																																									

Waking Temperature (grid of temperature values from 99 down through 96, with gradations 9–1 between each degree mark)

Cycle day	1	2	3	4	5	6	7	8	9	10	11	12	13	14	15	16	17	18	19	20	21	22	23	24	25	26	27	28	29	30	31	32	33	34	35	36	37	38	39	40	41
Peak Day																																									
Vaginal Sensation																																									

Cervix ● o O
         F M S

Mucus (BSE noted at cycle day 7)

Cycle day	1	2	3	4	5	6	7	8	9	10	11	12	13	14	15	16	17	18	19	20	21	22	23	24	25	26	27	28	29	30	31	32	33	34	35	36	37	38	39	40	41
Miscellaneous:																																									

A SUMMARY OF RULES FOR NOT GETTING PREGNANT

During the Menstrual Period

Because you can have mucus while you bleed or spot (and not be able to see or feel it), consider your period a fertile time during your first 12 charted cycles. Once you have had 12 ovulatory cycles in a row that are each 26 days or longer, you can consider yourself infertile Days 1 through 5. If you have had a cycle that is 25 days or shorter, you can consider yourself infertile Days 1 through 3.

Dry Day Rule

In a dry vagina, sperm can not live more than four hours. Once you notice mucus or wet vaginal sensation, you are fertile. Intercourse can lead to pregnancy. After the period (*and before ovulation*), you are infertile after 6 PM if you have been dry all day. The next day, you need to be dry all day again to call yourself infertile after 6 PM.

Peak Day Rule

The last day of wet mucus or wet vaginal sensation is called the Peak Day. Women usually ovulate on the Peak Day. When your mucus has dried up for several days, you have a sign from your body that your egg is gone for this cycle. You are infertile after 6 PM when you have four days in a row of mucus and vaginal sensation that are drier than your Peak Day.

Temperature Shift Rule

When your temperature goes up, count back six low temperatures; draw a coverline one tenth of a degree above the highest of these low temperatures. When your temperature is above your coverline for three days in a row, you are infertile after 6 PM on that third day.

If You Are Not Sure Whether You Are Fertile or Infertile

If you do not want a new pregnancy and you are not sure whether you are fertile or infertile, do not have intercourse. Consider yourself fertile until all of your signs tell you that you are infertile. If your mucus and temperature do not match, listen to the one that tells you that you are still fertile.

A SUMMARY OF WAYS TO HELP YOU GET PREGNANT

1. If your husband's sperm count is normal, have intercourse each day you have wet mucus or wet vaginal sensation. If his sperm count is low, have intercourse every other day that you have wetness. Either way, try to have intercourse on your Peak Day.

2. Try to make love on the first morning that your temperature jumps up.

3. Eat a healthy diet. Exercise regularly. Sleep in total darkness except around the days you have slippery mucus. (Read more about night lighting on pages 50-51.)

Fertility Cycle # _____

Start Date _____   # Days this cycle _____

Cycle day	1	2	3	4	5	6	7	8	9	10	11	12	13	14	15	16	17	18	19	20	21	22	23	24	25	26	27	28	29	30	31	32	33	34	35	36	37	38	39	40	41
Date																																									
Intercourse																																									
Time Temp Taken																																									
Temp count																																									

Waking Temperature (grid marked 99, 98, 97, 96 with subdivisions 9–1)

Cycle day	1	2	3	4	5	6	7	8	9	10	11	12	13	14	15	16	17	18	19	20	21	22	23	24	25	26	27	28	29	30	31	32	33	34	35	36	37	38	39	40	41
Peak Day																																									
Vaginal Sensation																																									
Cervix (● o O / F M S)																																									
Mucus						BSE																																			

Cycle day	1	2	3	4	5	6	7	8	9	10	11	12	13	14	15	16	17	18	19	20	21	22	23	24	25	26	27	28	29	30	31	32	33	34	35	36	37	38	39	40	41
Miscellaneous:																																									

A SUMMARY OF RULES FOR NOT GETTING PREGNANT

During the Menstrual Period

Because you can have mucus while you bleed or spot (and not be able to see or feel it), consider your period a fertile time during your first 12 charted cycles. Once you have had 12 ovulatory cycles in a row that are each 26 days or longer, you can consider yourself infertile Days 1 through 5. If you have had a cycle that is 25 days or shorter, you can consider yourself infertile Days 1 through 3.

Dry Day Rule

In a dry vagina, sperm can not live more than four hours. Once you notice mucus or wet vaginal sensation, you are fertile. Intercourse can lead to pregnancy. After the period (*and before ovulation*), you are infertile after 6 PM if you have been dry all day. The next day, you need to be dry all day again to call yourself infertile after 6 PM.

Peak Day Rule

The last day of wet mucus or wet vaginal sensation is called the Peak Day. Women usually ovulate on the Peak Day. When your mucus has dried up for several days, you have a sign from your body that your egg is gone for this cycle. You are infertile after 6 PM when you have four days in a row of mucus and vaginal sensation that are drier than your Peak Day.

Temperature Shift Rule

When your temperature goes up, count back six low temperatures; draw a coverline one tenth of a degree above the highest of these low temperatures. When your temperature is above your coverline for three days in a row, you are infertile after 6 PM on that third day.

If You Are Not Sure Whether You Are Fertile or Infertile

If you do not want a new pregnancy and you are not sure whether you are fertile or infertile, do not have intercourse. Consider yourself fertile until all of your signs tell you that you are infertile. If your mucus and temperature do not match, listen to the one that tells you that you are still fertile.

A SUMMARY OF WAYS TO HELP YOU GET PREGNANT

1. If your husband's sperm count is normal, have intercourse each day you have wet mucus or wet vaginal sensation. If his sperm count is low, have intercourse every other day that you have wetness. Either way, try to have intercourse on your Peak Day.

2. Try to make love on the first morning that your temperature jumps up.

3. Eat a healthy diet. Exercise regularly. Sleep in total darkness except around the days you have slippery mucus. (Read more about night lighting on pages 50-51.)

Fertility Cycle #_____

Start Date _____   # Days this cycle _____

Cycle day	1	2	3	4	5	6	7	8	9	10	11	12	13	14	15	16	17	18	19	20	21	22	23	24	25	26	27	28	29	30	31	32	33	34	35	36	37	38	39	40	41
Date																																									
Intercourse																																									
Time Temp Taken																																									
Temp count																																									

Waking Temperature (grid ranging 99, 98, 97, 96 with subdivisions 9–1)

Cycle day	1	2	3	4	5	6	7	8	9	10	11	12	13	14	15	16	17	18	19	20	21	22	23	24	25	26	27	28	29	30	31	32	33	34	35	36	37	38	39	40	41
Peak Day																																									
Vaginal Sensation																																									

Cervix: ● o O / F M S

Mucus

(Note: BSE marked at Cycle day 7)

Cycle day	1	2	3	4	5	6	7	8	9	10	11	12	13	14	15	16	17	18	19	20	21	22	23	24	25	26	27	28	29	30	31	32	33	34	35	36	37	38	39	40	41
Miscellaneous:																																									

www.GardenofFertility.com

A SUMMARY OF RULES FOR NOT GETTING PREGNANT

During the Menstrual Period

Because you can have mucus while you bleed or spot (and not be able to see or feel it), consider your period a fertile time during your first 12 charted cycles. Once you have had 12 ovulatory cycles in a row that are each 26 days or longer, you can consider yourself infertile Days 1 through 5. If you have had a cycle that is 25 days or shorter, you can consider yourself infertile Days 1 through 3.

Dry Day Rule

In a dry vagina, sperm can not live more than four hours. Once you notice mucus or wet vaginal sensation, you are fertile. Intercourse can lead to pregnancy. After the period (*and before ovulation*), you are infertile after 6 PM if you have been dry all day. The next day, you need to be dry all day again to call yourself infertile after 6 PM.

Peak Day Rule

The last day of wet mucus or wet vaginal sensation is called the Peak Day. Women usually ovulate on the Peak Day. When your mucus has dried up for several days, you have a sign from your body that your egg is gone for this cycle. You are infertile after 6 PM when you have four days in a row of mucus and vaginal sensation that are drier than your Peak Day.

Temperature Shift Rule

When your temperature goes up, count back six low temperatures; draw a coverline one tenth of a degree above the highest of these low temperatures. When your temperature is above your coverline for three days in a row, you are infertile after 6 PM on that third day.

If You Are Not Sure Whether You Are Fertile or Infertile

If you do not want a new pregnancy and you are not sure whether you are fertile or infertile, do not have intercourse. Consider yourself fertile until all of your signs tell you that you are infertile. If your mucus and temperature do not match, listen to the one that tells you that you are still fertile.

A SUMMARY OF WAYS TO HELP YOU GET PREGNANT

1. If your husband's sperm count is normal, have intercourse each day you have wet mucus or wet vaginal sensation. If his sperm count is low, have intercourse every other day that you have wetness. Either way, try to have intercourse on your Peak Day.

2. Try to make love on the first morning that your temperature jumps up.

3. Eat a healthy diet. Exercise regularly. Sleep in total darkness except around the days you have slippery mucus. (Read more about night lighting on pages 50-51.)

Fertility Cycle #_____

Start Date _____   # Days this cycle _____

Cycle day	1	2	3	4	5	6	7	8	9	10	11	12	13	14	15	16	17	18	19	20	21	22	23	24	25	26	27	28	29	30	31	32	33	34	35	36	37	38	39	40	41
Date																																									
Intercourse																																									
Time Temp Taken																																									
Temp count																																									

Waking Temperature grid (99 / 98 / 97 / 96 ranges with numbered subdivisions 9–1)

Cycle day	1	2	3	4	5	6	7	8	9	10	11	12	13	14	15	16	17	18	19	20	21	22	23	24	25	26	27	28	29	30	31	32	33	34	35	36	37	38	39	40	41
Peak Day																																									
Vaginal Sensation																																									
Cervix ● o O / F M S																																									
Mucus							BSE																																		

Cycle day	1	2	3	4	5	6	7	8	9	10	11	12	13	14	15	16	17	18	19	20	21	22	23	24	25	26	27	28	29	30	31	32	33	34	35	36	37	38	39	40	41
Miscellaneous:																																									

A SUMMARY OF RULES FOR NOT GETTING PREGNANT

During the Menstrual Period

Because you can have mucus while you bleed or spot (and not be able to see or feel it), consider your period a fertile time during your first 12 charted cycles. Once you have had 12 ovulatory cycles in a row that are each 26 days or longer, you can consider yourself infertile Days 1 through 5. If you have had a cycle that is 25 days or shorter, you can consider yourself infertile Days 1 through 3.

Dry Day Rule

In a dry vagina, sperm can not live more than four hours. Once you notice mucus or wet vaginal sensation, you are fertile. Intercourse can lead to pregnancy. After the period (*and before ovulation*), you are infertile after 6 PM if you have been dry all day. The next day, you need to be dry all day again to call yourself infertile after 6 PM.

Peak Day Rule

The last day of wet mucus or wet vaginal sensation is called the Peak Day. Women usually ovulate on the Peak Day. When your mucus has dried up for several days, you have a sign from your body that your egg is gone for this cycle. You are infertile after 6 PM when you have four days in a row of mucus and vaginal sensation that are drier than your Peak Day.

Temperature Shift Rule

When your temperature goes up, count back six low temperatures; draw a coverline one tenth of a degree above the highest of these low temperatures. When your temperature is above your coverline for three days in a row, you are infertile after 6 PM on that third day.

If You Are Not Sure Whether You Are Fertile or Infertile

If you do not want a new pregnancy and you are not sure whether you are fertile or infertile, do not have intercourse. Consider yourself fertile until all of your signs tell you that you are infertile. If your mucus and temperature do not match, listen to the one that tells you that you are still fertile.

A SUMMARY OF WAYS TO HELP YOU GET PREGNANT

1. If your husband's sperm count is normal, have intercourse each day you have wet mucus or wet vaginal sensation. If his sperm count is low, have intercourse every other day that you have wetness. Either way, try to have intercourse on your Peak Day.

2. Try to make love on the first morning that your temperature jumps up.

3. Eat a healthy diet. Exercise regularly. Sleep in total darkness except around the days you have slippery mucus. (Read more about night lighting on pages 50-51.)

Fertility Cycle #_____

Start Date _____

Days this cycle _____

Cycle day	1	2	3	4	5	6	7	8	9	10	11	12	13	14	15	16	17	18	19	20	21	22	23	24	25	26	27	28	29	30	31	32	33	34	35	36	37	38	39	40	41
Date																																									
Intercourse																																									
Time Temp Taken																																									
Temp count																																									

Waking Temperature (scale 99 → 96 degrees with tenths 9–1 for each)

Cycle day	1	2	3	4	5	6	7	8	9	10	11	12	13	14	15	16	17	18	19	20	21	22	23	24	25	26	27	28	29	30	31	32	33	34	35	36	37	38	39	40	41
Peak Day																																									
Vaginal Sensation																																									

Cervix: ● o O / F M S

Mucus

(BSE marked on Cycle day 7)

Cycle day	1	2	3	4	5	6	7	8	9	10	11	12	13	14	15	16	17	18	19	20	21	22	23	24	25	26	27	28	29	30	31	32	33	34	35	36	37	38	39	40	41
Miscellaneous:																																									

A SUMMARY OF RULES FOR NOT GETTING PREGNANT

During the Menstrual Period

Because you can have mucus while you bleed or spot (and not be able to see or feel it), consider your period a fertile time during your first 12 charted cycles. Once you have had 12 ovulatory cycles in a row that are each 26 days or longer, you can consider yourself infertile Days 1 through 5. If you have had a cycle that is 25 days or shorter, you can consider yourself infertile Days 1 through 3.

Dry Day Rule

In a dry vagina, sperm can not live more than four hours. Once you notice mucus or wet vaginal sensation, you are fertile. Intercourse can lead to pregnancy. After the period (*and before ovulation*), you are infertile after 6 PM if you have been dry all day. The next day, you need to be dry all day again to call yourself infertile after 6 PM.

Peak Day Rule

The last day of wet mucus or wet vaginal sensation is called the Peak Day. Women usually ovulate on the Peak Day. When your mucus has dried up for several days, you have a sign from your body that your egg is gone for this cycle. You are infertile after 6 PM when you have four days in a row of mucus and vaginal sensation that are drier than your Peak Day.

Temperature Shift Rule

When your temperature goes up, count back six low temperatures; draw a coverline one tenth of a degree above the highest of these low temperatures. When your temperature is above your coverline for three days in a row, you are infertile after 6 PM on that third day.

If You Are Not Sure Whether You Are Fertile or Infertile

If you do not want a new pregnancy and you are not sure whether you are fertile or infertile, do not have intercourse. Consider yourself fertile until all of your signs tell you that you are infertile. If your mucus and temperature do not match, listen to the one that tells you that you are still fertile.

A SUMMARY OF WAYS TO HELP YOU GET PREGNANT

1. If your husband's sperm count is normal, have intercourse each day you have wet mucus or wet vaginal sensation. If his sperm count is low, have intercourse every other day that you have wetness. Either way, try to have intercourse on your Peak Day.

2. Try to make love on the first morning that your temperature jumps up.

3. Eat a healthy diet. Exercise regularly. Sleep in total darkness except around the days you have slippery mucus. (Read more about night lighting on pages 50-51.)

Fertility Cycle #_____

Start Date _____   # Days this cycle _____

Cycle day	1	2	3	4	5	6	7	8	9	10	11	12	13	14	15	16	17	18	19	20	21	22	23	24	25	26	27	28	29	30	31	32	33	34	35	36	37	38	39	40	41
Date																																									
Intercourse																																									
Time Temp Taken																																									
Temp count																																									

Waking Temperature (grid of temperature values from 96.9 up through 99 for each cycle day 1–41)

Cycle day	1	2	3	4	5	6	7	8	9	10	11	12	13	14	15	16	17	18	19	20	21	22	23	24	25	26	27	28	29	30	31	32	33	34	35	36	37	38	39	40	41
Peak Day																																									
Vaginal Sensation																																									
Cervix (● o ◯ / F M S)																																									
Mucus							BSE																																		

Cycle day	1	2	3	4	5	6	7	8	9	10	11	12	13	14	15	16	17	18	19	20	21	22	23	24	25	26	27	28	29	30	31	32	33	34	35	36	37	38	39	40	41
Miscellaneous:																																									

www.GardenofFertility.com

A SUMMARY OF RULES FOR NOT GETTING PREGNANT

During the Menstrual Period

Because you can have mucus while you bleed or spot (and not be able to see or feel it), consider your period a fertile time during your first 12 charted cycles. Once you have had 12 ovulatory cycles in a row that are each 26 days or longer, you can consider yourself infertile Days 1 through 5. If you have had a cycle that is 25 days or shorter, you can consider yourself infertile Days 1 through 3.

Dry Day Rule

In a dry vagina, sperm can not live more than four hours. Once you notice mucus or wet vaginal sensation, you are fertile. Intercourse can lead to pregnancy. After the period (*and before ovulation*), you are infertile after 6 PM if you have been dry all day. The next day, you need to be dry all day again to call yourself infertile after 6 PM.

Peak Day Rule

The last day of wet mucus or wet vaginal sensation is called the Peak Day. Women usually ovulate on the Peak Day. When your mucus has dried up for several days, you have a sign from your body that your egg is gone for this cycle. You are infertile after 6 PM when you have four days in a row of mucus and vaginal sensation that are drier than your Peak Day.

Temperature Shift Rule

When your temperature goes up, count back six low temperatures; draw a coverline one tenth of a degree above the highest of these low temperatures. When your temperature is above your coverline for three days in a row, you are infertile after 6 PM on that third day.

If You Are Not Sure Whether You Are Fertile or Infertile

If you do not want a new pregnancy and you are not sure whether you are fertile or infertile, do not have intercourse. Consider yourself fertile until all of your signs tell you that you are infertile. If your mucus and temperature do not match, listen to the one that tells you that you are still fertile.

A SUMMARY OF WAYS TO HELP YOU GET PREGNANT

1. If your husband's sperm count is normal, have intercourse each day you have wet mucus or wet vaginal sensation. If his sperm count is low, have intercourse every other day that you have wetness. Either way, try to have intercourse on your Peak Day.

2. Try to make love on the first morning that your temperature jumps up.

3. Eat a healthy diet. Exercise regularly. Sleep in total darkness except around the days you have slippery mucus. (Read more about night lighting on pages 50-51.)

Fertility Cycle # _____

Start Date _____   # Days this cycle _____

Cycle day	1	2	3	4	5	6	7	8	9	10	11	12	13	14	15	16	17	18	19	20	21	22	23	24	25	26	27	28	29	30	31	32	33	34	35	36	37	38	39	40	41
Date																																									
Intercourse																																									
Time Temp Taken																																									
Temp count																																									

Waking Temperature — temperature grid (99 down to 96.9), spanning columns for each cycle day.

Cycle day	1	2	3	4	5	6	7	8	9	10	11	12	13	14	15	16	17	18	19	20	21	22	23	24	25	26	27	28	29	30	31	32	33	34	35	36	37	38	39	40	41
Peak Day																																									
Vaginal Sensation																																									

Cervix: ● o O / F M S

Mucus: (BSE noted at cycle day 7)

Cycle day	1	2	3	4	5	6	7	8	9	10	11	12	13	14	15	16	17	18	19	20	21	22	23	24	25	26	27	28	29	30	31	32	33	34	35	36	37	38	39	40	41
Miscellaneous:																																									

www.GardenofFertility.com

A SUMMARY OF RULES FOR NOT GETTING PREGNANT

During the Menstrual Period

Because you can have mucus while you bleed or spot (and not be able to see or feel it), consider your period a fertile time during your first 12 charted cycles. Once you have had 12 ovulatory cycles in a row that are each 26 days or longer, you can consider yourself infertile Days 1 through 5. If you have had a cycle that is 25 days or shorter, you can consider yourself infertile Days 1 through 3.

Dry Day Rule

In a dry vagina, sperm can not live more than four hours. Once you notice mucus or wet vaginal sensation, you are fertile. Intercourse can lead to pregnancy. After the period (*and before ovulation*), you are infertile after 6 PM if you have been dry all day. The next day, you need to be dry all day again to call yourself infertile after 6 PM.

Peak Day Rule

The last day of wet mucus or wet vaginal sensation is called the Peak Day. Women usually ovulate on the Peak Day. When your mucus has dried up for several days, you have a sign from your body that your egg is gone for this cycle. You are infertile after 6 PM when you have four days in a row of mucus and vaginal sensation that are drier than your Peak Day.

Temperature Shift Rule

When your temperature goes up, count back six low temperatures; draw a coverline one tenth of a degree above the highest of these low temperatures. When your temperature is above your coverline for three days in a row, you are infertile after 6 PM on that third day.

If You Are Not Sure Whether You Are Fertile or Infertile

If you do not want a new pregnancy and you are not sure whether you are fertile or infertile, do not have intercourse. Consider yourself fertile until all of your signs tell you that you are infertile. If your mucus and temperature do not match, listen to the one that tells you that you are still fertile.

A SUMMARY OF WAYS TO HELP YOU GET PREGNANT

1. If your husband's sperm count is normal, have intercourse each day you have wet mucus or wet vaginal sensation. If his sperm count is low, have intercourse every other day that you have wetness. Either way, try to have intercourse on your Peak Day.

2. Try to make love on the first morning that your temperature jumps up.
3. Eat a healthy diet. Exercise regularly. Sleep in total darkness except around the days you have slippery mucus. (Read more about night lighting on pages 50-51.)

Fertility Cycle #_____

Start Date _____   # Days this cycle _____

Cycle day	1	2	3	4	5	6	7	8	9	10	11	12	13	14	15	16	17	18	19	20	21	22	23	24	25	26	27	28	29	30	31	32	33	34	35	36	37	38	39	40	41
Date																																									
Intercourse																																									
Time Temp Taken																																									
Temp count																																									

Waking Temperature (grid from 99 down to 96⁹ for each cycle day 1–41)

Cycle day	1	2	3	4	5	6	7	8	9	10	11	12	13	14	15	16	17	18	19	20	21	22	23	24	25	26	27	28	29	30	31	32	33	34	35	36	37	38	39	40	41
Peak Day																																									
Vaginal Sensation																																									
Cervix ● ○ ◯ F M S																																									
Mucus							BSE																																		

Cycle day	1	2	3	4	5	6	7	8	9	10	11	12	13	14	15	16	17	18	19	20	21	22	23	24	25	26	27	28	29	30	31	32	33	34	35	36	37	38	39	40	41
Miscellaneous:																																									

www.GardenofFertility.com

A SUMMARY OF RULES FOR NOT GETTING PREGNANT

During the Menstrual Period

Because you can have mucus while you bleed or spot (and not be able to see or feel it), consider your period a fertile time during your first 12 charted cycles. Once you have had 12 ovulatory cycles in a row that are each 26 days or longer, you can consider yourself infertile Days 1 through 5. If you have had a cycle that is 25 days or shorter, you can consider yourself infertile Days 1 through 3.

Dry Day Rule

In a dry vagina, sperm can not live more than four hours. Once you notice mucus or wet vaginal sensation, you are fertile. Intercourse can lead to pregnancy. After the period (*and before ovulation*), you are infertile after 6 PM if you have been dry all day. The next day, you need to be dry all day again to call yourself infertile after 6 PM.

Peak Day Rule

The last day of wet mucus or wet vaginal sensation is called the Peak Day. Women usually ovulate on the Peak Day. When your mucus has dried up for several days, you have a sign from your body that your egg is gone for this cycle. You are infertile after 6 PM when you have four days in a row of mucus and vaginal sensation that are drier than your Peak Day.

Temperature Shift Rule

When your temperature goes up, count back six low temperatures; draw a coverline one tenth of a degree above the highest of these low temperatures. When your temperature is above your coverline for three days in a row, you are infertile after 6 PM on that third day.

If You Are Not Sure Whether You Are Fertile or Infertile

If you do not want a new pregnancy and you are not sure whether you are fertile or infertile, do not have intercourse. Consider yourself fertile until all of your signs tell you that you are infertile. If your mucus and temperature do not match, listen to the one that tells you that you are still fertile.

A SUMMARY OF WAYS TO HELP YOU GET PREGNANT

1. If your husband's sperm count is normal, have intercourse each day you have wet mucus or wet vaginal sensation. If his sperm count is low, have intercourse every other day that you have wetness. Either way, try to have intercourse on your Peak Day.

2. Try to make love on the first morning that your temperature jumps up.

3. Eat a healthy diet. Exercise regularly. Sleep in total darkness except around the days you have slippery mucus. (Read more about night lighting on pages 50-51.)

Fertility Cycle #_____

Start Date _____   # Days this cycle _____

Cycle day	1	2	3	4	5	6	7	8	9	10	11	12	13	14	15	16	17	18	19	20	21	22	23	24	25	26	27	28	29	30	31	32	33	34	35	36	37	38	39	40	41
Date																																									
Intercourse																																									
Time Temp Taken																																									
Temp count																																									

Waking Temperature

(Temperature grid: rows 99, 98, 97, 96 each with sub-gradations 9–1, across cycle days 1–41)

Cycle day	1	2	3	4	5	6	7	8	9	10	11	12	13	14	15	16	17	18	19	20	21	22	23	24	25	26	27	28	29	30	31	32	33	34	35	36	37	38	39	40	41
Peak Day																																									
Vaginal Sensation																																									
Cervix																																									

Cervix legend: ● o O / F M S

Mucus

(In mucus column at cycle day 7: BSE)

Cycle day	1	2	3	4	5	6	7	8	9	10	11	12	13	14	15	16	17	18	19	20	21	22	23	24	25	26	27	28	29	30	31	32	33	34	35	36	37	38	39	40	41
Miscellaneous:																																									

A SUMMARY OF RULES FOR NOT GETTING PREGNANT

During the Menstrual Period

Because you can have mucus while you bleed or spot (and not be able to see or feel it), consider your period a fertile time during your first 12 charted cycles. Once you have had 12 ovulatory cycles in a row that are each 26 days or longer, you can consider yourself infertile Days 1 through 5. If you have had a cycle that is 25 days or shorter, you can consider yourself infertile Days 1 through 3.

Dry Day Rule

In a dry vagina, sperm can not live more than four hours. Once you notice mucus or wet vaginal sensation, you are fertile. Intercourse can lead to pregnancy. After the period (*and before ovulation*), you are infertile after 6 PM if you have been dry all day. The next day, you need to be dry all day again to call yourself infertile after 6 PM.

Peak Day Rule

The last day of wet mucus or wet vaginal sensation is called the Peak Day. Women usually ovulate on the Peak Day. When your mucus has dried up for several days, you have a sign from your body that your egg is gone for this cycle. You are infertile after 6 PM when you have four days in a row of mucus and vaginal sensation that are drier than your Peak Day.

Temperature Shift Rule

When your temperature goes up, count back six low temperatures; draw a coverline one tenth of a degree above the highest of these low temperatures. When your temperature is above your coverline for three days in a row, you are infertile after 6 PM on that third day.

If You Are Not Sure Whether You Are Fertile or Infertile

If you do not want a new pregnancy and you are not sure whether you are fertile or infertile, do not have intercourse. Consider yourself fertile until all of your signs tell you that you are infertile. If your mucus and temperature do not match, listen to the one that tells you that you are still fertile.

A SUMMARY OF WAYS TO HELP YOU GET PREGNANT

1. If your husband's sperm count is normal, have intercourse each day you have wet mucus or wet vaginal sensation. If his sperm count is low, have intercourse every other day that you have wetness. Either way, try to have intercourse on your Peak Day.

2. Try to make love on the first morning that your temperature jumps up.

3. Eat a healthy diet. Exercise regularly. Sleep in total darkness except around the days you have slippery mucus. (Read more about night lighting on pages 50-51.)

Fertility Cycle #_____

Start Date _____   # Days this cycle _____

Cycle day	1	2	3	4	5	6	7	8	9	10	11	12	13	14	15	16	17	18	19	20	21	22	23	24	25	26	27	28	29	30	31	32	33	34	35	36	37	38	39	40	41
Date																																									
Intercourse																																									
Time Temp Taken																																									
Temp count																																									

Waking Temperature (grid of values 99 through 96, with tenths 9–1)

Cycle day	1	2	3	4	5	6	7	8	9	10	11	12	13	14	15	16	17	18	19	20	21	22	23	24	25	26	27	28	29	30	31	32	33	34	35	36	37	38	39	40	41
Peak Day																																									
Vaginal Sensation																																									
Cervix (● o O / F M S)																																									
Mucus						BSE																																			

Cycle day	1	2	3	4	5	6	7	8	9	10	11	12	13	14	15	16	17	18	19	20	21	22	23	24	25	26	27	28	29	30	31	32	33	34	35	36	37	38	39	40	41
Miscellaneous:																																									

www.GardenofFertility.com

A SUMMARY OF RULES FOR NOT GETTING PREGNANT

During the Menstrual Period

Because you can have mucus while you bleed or spot (and not be able to see or feel it), consider your period a fertile time during your first 12 charted cycles. Once you have had 12 ovulatory cycles in a row that are each 26 days or longer, you can consider yourself infertile Days 1 through 5. If you have had a cycle that is 25 days or shorter, you can consider yourself infertile Days 1 through 3.

Dry Day Rule

In a dry vagina, sperm can not live more than four hours. Once you notice mucus or wet vaginal sensation, you are fertile. Intercourse can lead to pregnancy. After the period (*and before ovulation*), you are infertile after 6 PM if you have been dry all day. The next day, you need to be dry all day again to call yourself infertile after 6 PM.

Peak Day Rule

The last day of wet mucus or wet vaginal sensation is called the Peak Day. Women usually ovulate on the Peak Day. When your mucus has dried up for several days, you have a sign from your body that your egg is gone for this cycle. You are infertile after 6 PM when you have four days in a row of mucus and vaginal sensation that are drier than your Peak Day.

Temperature Shift Rule

When your temperature goes up, count back six low temperatures; draw a coverline one tenth of a degree above the highest of these low temperatures. When your temperature is above your coverline for three days in a row, you are infertile after 6 PM on that third day.

If You Are Not Sure Whether You Are Fertile or Infertile

If you do not want a new pregnancy and you are not sure whether you are fertile or infertile, do not have intercourse. Consider yourself fertile until all of your signs tell you that you are infertile. If your mucus and temperature do not match, listen to the one that tells you that you are still fertile.

A SUMMARY OF WAYS TO HELP YOU GET PREGNANT

1. If your husband's sperm count is normal, have intercourse each day you have wet mucus or wet vaginal sensation. If his sperm count is low, have intercourse every other day that you have wetness. Either way, try to have intercourse on your Peak Day.

2. Try to make love on the first morning that your temperature jumps up.

3. Eat a healthy diet. Exercise regularly. Sleep in total darkness except around the days you have slippery mucus. (Read more about night lighting on pages 50-51.)

Fertility Cycle #_____

Start Date _____   # Days this cycle _____

Cycle day	1	2	3	4	5	6	7	8	9	10	11	12	13	14	15	16	17	18	19	20	21	22	23	24	25	26	27	28	29	30	31	32	33	34	35	36	37	38	39	40	41
Date																																									
Intercourse																																									
Time Temp Taken																																									
Temp count																																									

Waking Temperature (degrees marked 99, 98, 97, 96 with subdivisions 9–1 for each row, repeated across all 41 cycle day columns)

Cycle day	1	2	3	4	5	6	7	8	9	10	11	12	13	14	15	16	17	18	19	20	21	22	23	24	25	26	27	28	29	30	31	32	33	34	35	36	37	38	39	40	41
Peak Day																																									
Vaginal Sensation																																									
Cervix (● o O / F M S)																																									
Mucus							BSE																																		

Cycle day	1	2	3	4	5	6	7	8	9	10	11	12	13	14	15	16	17	18	19	20	21	22	23	24	25	26	27	28	29	30	31	32	33	34	35	36	37	38	39	40	41
Miscellaneous:																																									

www.GardenofFertility.com

To purchase a copy of *Honoring Our Cycles*, send a check for $17.00
($12 for the book, plus $5 for shipping and handling) to:

New Trends Publishing
401 Kings Highway
Winona Lake, IN 46590

To purchase a case of 24 books at 50% off plus shipping
contact the publisher at
newtrends@kconline.com or call 877.707.1776.
For international orders, call 574.268.2601.